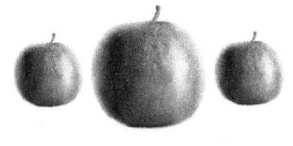

APPLE-A-DAY BOOKS

www.AppleADayBooks.com

100 Questions EVERY Patient Should Ask BEFORE Surgery

1st Edition, 2010

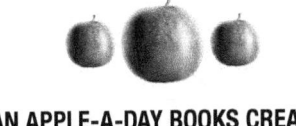

AN APPLE-A-DAY BOOKS CREATION

100 Questions Every Patient Should Ask Before Surgery

Published by Apple A Day Books/CreateSpace LLC.
Copyright © 2010 Apple A Day Books

Printed in the United States of America

First Edition, 2010

Library of Congress Cataloging-in-Publication Data

ISBN-10: 1453691375
EAN-13: 9781453691373

For more information, please visit
www.AppleADayBooks.com

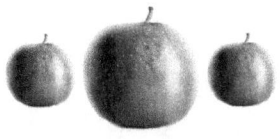

ABOUT APPLE-A-DAY BOOKS

Apple-A-Day Books was created by Ognjen "Ogi" Visnjevac and Frederick Ma as an official medical student promotion and publication company.

Realizing the incredible value of the too-often squandered eager student mind, *Apple-A-Day Books'* goal is to create publications for three purposes: (1) to improve medical and health education; (2) to provide new and innovative public health solutions; and (3) to inspire students to do more, to advance their careers, and to take responsibility as leaders in healthcare within their own communities.

For more information about *Apple-A-Day Books*, visit:
www.AppleADayBooks.com

OTHER TITLES FROM APPLE-A-DAY BOOKS

Community Education Division

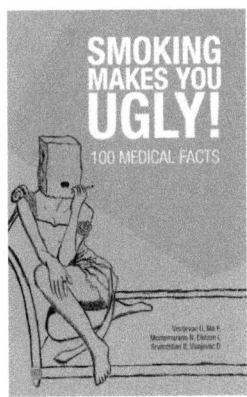

Smoking Makes You Ugly!
100 Medical Facts, 1st Edition

ISBN: 1449990614

Medical School Education Division

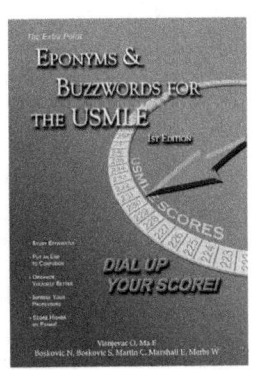

The Extra Point: Eponyms & Buzzwords
for the USMLE, 1st Edition

ISBN: 1449985289

EDITORS-IN-CHIEF

OGNJEN "OGI" VISNJEVAC, MS-IV
St. George's University School of Medicine

FREDERICK MA, MS-IV
St. George's University School of Medicine

ILLUSTRATOR

IVA HOLOVAC
Graphic Designer, www.ivaholovac.com

COPY EDITOR

MARKO PERKOVIC
Victoria, British Columbia

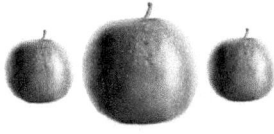

This book is dually dedicated:

First, to the family and friends who continue to support and teach us.

Second, to our past patients and to every patient who is about to undergo surgery, along with their friends and families; we hope this book helps you before you go to the operating room.

A Note For All:

The basic premise of any surgical specialty:

All decisions made to pursue a surgical intervention result from an understanding of the balance of risks versus benefits. The risks include those risks of the procedure (complications, infections, etc) as well as the risks of NOT performing the operation. The benefits include an evaluation of the magnitude of the benefit (example: the ability to wiggle a toe versus the ability to stand on that foot) and the likelihood of those benefits.

ACKNOWLEDGMENTS

We would like to thank the following people for their help, ideas, inputs, and support throughout the writing and development of this book:

Our Patients,
Dr. M. Daniels, Dr. R. Foege, Dr. J. Frederic,
Dr. S. Reitzen, T. Krunic, Dr. A. Winkler, Dr. T. Witschi,
Family Visnjevac, and all of the friends and family
who continue to support our efforts.

TABLE OF CONTENTS

DISCLAIMER

The contents presented herein, such as text, graphics, and other material ("Content") published in this book, *100 Questions Every Patient Should Ask Before Surgery* ("Book") or located at appleadaybooks.com and its subdomains or aliases ("Website") are for informational purposes only. The Content is not intended as a substitute for professional medical/dental advice, diagnosis, or treatment. Always seek the advice of your physician, dental professional, or other qualified health provider with any questions you may have regarding a medical/dental condition. Never disregard professional medical/dental advice or delay in seeking it because of Content found herein.

If you have a medical/dental emergency, call your physician/dentist or 911 immediately. Apple-A-Day Books, its employees, the authors, editors, illustrators, and other acknowledged parties, or others appearing on the Website at the invitation of Apple A Day Books ("Contributors") do not recommend or endorse any specific third-party tests, physicians, products, procedures, opinions, or other information found within this book. Reliance on any information provided in this Book or this Website by the Contributors or other visitors to the Website is solely at your own risk.

Reading the information on this Website does not create a physician-patient relationship. If you need specific medical advice please seek a professional who is licensed or knowledgeable in that area.

Reading the information on this Website does not create a physician-patient relationship. If you need specific medical advice please seek a professional who is licensed or knowledgeable in that area.

This document cannot be used for any legal purposes.

GLOSSARY OF TERMS

Acute respiratory distress syndrome (ARDS) – a severe lung condition that is characterized by inflammation of the lung tissue and impaired oxygen perfusion. It may lead to multiple organ failure and has several causes, including severe infections, pneumonia, and/ or multiple blood transfusions. Most patients require intubation and assisted ventilation.

Coagulopathy – a defect in the body's circulatory or hematopoietic systems' ability to form and regulate blood clot formation. This may be an inherited disorder that may include hemophilia, or may be acquired through medications, severe infections, or organ dysfunctions.

Cardiac catheterization – a diagnostic and interventional procedure involving insertion of a catheter into the heart and its related vessels. Uses for cardiac catheterization includes patients with heart attacks, investigation of potential heart disease, or assessing patients prior to surgery.

CT Scan (Computer tomography) – a noninvasive imagine technique that uses computer processing to generate a 3-D image from a series of 2-D X-ray images.

Echocardiogram – an ultrasound used to visualize potential heart defects and estimate the function of a heart. This may be done by applying the ultrasound on the chest wall (Transthoracic echocardiogram) or through inserting the ultrasound device inside the esophagus (Transesophageal echocardiogram), which will require sedation of the patient.

Elective surgery – an operation or procedure that is not a medical emergency.

Heart sounds – a sound that is heard with a stethoscope when listening to the heart. This sound is created due to turbulence or irregular blood flow within the heart. Heart sounds may have different intensities and different anatomical positions, and may be both normal or abnormal depending on the individual.

Healthcare proxy – someone you appoint by law to assist in making decisions for you in case you become mentally incapacitated.

Intravenous (IV) contrast – special dyes (radiocontrast materials containing radiation) that are injected into a patient's vein to help doctors see the internal organs and structures when using X-ray, CT scans, or MRI. Different contrast substances are used for each type of imaging modality.

Intraveous (IV) medication - a form of administering medication into the patient's veins that provides quicker delivery and greater effectiveness of the medication.

Laparoscopic surgery – surgery performed with minimally invasive techniques that does not require big incisions. Typically there will be multiple small incisions for placement of surgical tools and miniature cameras to visualize the inside of the body, where surgery will be performed.

Magnetic Resonance Imaging (MRI) – a noninvasive imaging technique that visualizes the body through the use of a powerful magnetic field to align hydrogen atoms in our body. This imaging modality has much higher contrast than ultrasound, x-ray, and CT scans. It may be used to take static or dynamic (moving) images. Individuals with metals in their body usually cannot receive an MRI. Tracheal Intubation – a method of providing ventilatory support that requires the placement of a flexible long tube down the throat. The procedure assists breathing for patients who are very ill, injured, or may not have the ability to breath on their own.

Palliative care – a form a medical care that concentrates on reducing the severity of symptoms of a disease and strives to bring comfort for a patient. The goal is to prevent suffering for a patient and this form of care may be applied for patients who may have incurable medical conditions.

Pulmonary edema – a condition where the lung tissue has too much fluid in it, limiting the lungs' ability to perfuse oxygen.

Pulmonary embolism – a blockage in the arteries that supply blood to the lungs to be re-oxygenated. It may be due to a blood clot or particles that may block lung artery circulation. This is an emergency and may be fatal to some individuals depending on the anatomical position of the blockage. Symptoms include cough, shortness of breath, and chest pain.

Ultrasound/Sonography – a noninvasive imaging technique based on ultrasound or acoustic energies to visualize internal body structures. This technique can be applied to visualize several different organs including the heart (echocardiogram), uterus, kidney, liver, gall bladder, etc.

X-ray film – a form of electromagnetic radiation imaging, using x-rays to create an image and visualize the body internally. Due to the low resolution and quality of the X-ray, not all medical conditions may be diagnosed solely by an X-ray and may require higher resolution imaging techniques.

EMERGENCY SURGERY

// See Disclaimer on page 1 of this book before reading this chapter.

Authors:

ANDREI KOMOROWSKY, MS-IV
St. George's University School of Medicine

OGNJEN "OGI" VISNJEVAC, MS-IV
St. George's University School of Medicine

Editors:

FAUSTO VINCES, D.O., FACS
Director of Trauma Services
Lutheran Medical Center, Brooklyn, NY

MATTHEW S. FRIEDMAN, M.D.
Resident Physician, Emergency Medicine Residency Training Program
Mount Sinai School of Medicine
Mount Sinai Medical Center, NY, NY

Q What blood type am I? Do the emergency room doctors know?

An individual's blood type refers to the specific chemical coat (an "antigen") on the surface of the red blood cells. There are four major blood types (Blood types A, B, AB and O), each of which can have a "negative" or "positive" subtype (examples: A-negative, O-positive).

This is relevant in that certain blood types also possess antibodies against other types of blood groups, meaning that their bodies' immune systems would react to a transfusion of blood from a different blood type by destroying all of the different or "foreign" blood. If there is an incompatibility between the donor's blood type and the receiver's, there is potential for the transfused red blood cells to burst, leading to kidney failure, shock or even death. In situations of severe blood loss, blood transfusions are often required to resuscitate the patient so it is extremely important to have a good match between the donor's and recipient's blood types.

If you do not know your blood type, you could ask your physician. In an emergency situation at a hospital, a sample of your blood would urgently be sent to the lab in order to find out your blood type just in case you need a transfusion. In a situation when a transfusion is required so urgently that there is no time to send a sample of blood to the lab, type O-negative blood is given because O-negative blood is safe for almost everyone. O-negative is rare, however, so it is better to receive blood matched to your blood type.

Q Does the hospital need to know about my religious views?

In cases of trauma whereby an individual has lost a substantial amount of blood, it may be necessary to resuscitate him or her using both intravenous (IV) fluids and blood transfusions. If your religious views, such as those of Jehovah's witnesses, prevent you from receiving blood products, feel free to inform the medical team that you do not wish to be given blood products. Before making such a decision, it is important to know the majority of clinical evidence shows that a trauma patient's outcome is usually significantly worse when necessary red blood cell or platelet transfusions are withheld.

In the past some people have also had concerns about blood borne diseases such as HIV and Hepatitis B or C being transmitted in blood products. Over the past two decades, however, blood has been continuously and rigorously tested for these viruses and more, so the chance of acquiring such an infection from a blood transfusion is exceedingly low.

It will also be important to differentiate between blood, red blood cells, platelets, albumin, clotting factors, and plasma (the fluid red blood cells float in). Some people do not want any of these blood products, but some choose to avoid only one or two of these, like avoiding red blood cells only while being comfortable with the notion of receiving platelets, plasma, clotting factors, or albumin.

Bloodless surgery is a technique used by some surgeons for elective surgery, whereby the patient donates his or her own blood ahead of time so that this blood may be used as a transfusion during the procedure. Intravenous (IV) fluids can also sometimes be used to increase the volume of fluid inside blood vessels in situations of blood loss.

Many cultures have their own specific practices regarding healthcare, including those specific to patients who pass away. Most hospitals try to accommodate religious requests; so do not hesitate to inform the hospital staff of your own personal needs.

For example, autopsies are often necessary to determine the cause of death, which may have both medical and legal implications, but the families of the recently deceased have the right to object to an autopsy based on religious views. Following such an objection, the families are typically given an opportunity to hire an attorney and to present their objection to a Court that will determine whether an autopsy will be performed. If there is a suspicious or traumatic death, the Judge may be more inclined not to grant the request, although the specific laws may vary state-by-state and country-by-country.

Q Who will be in charge of making decisions on my behalf if I cannot do so myself?

In emergency situations like car accidents or heart attacks, the patient is often either unconscious or conscious but unable to make his or her own decisions. Such patients need to designate someone as a health care proxy, typically a spouse or family member, who will be chosen to make medical/legal decisions in situations where the patient does not have the capacity to make them. This is particularly common in cases of head trauma, neurological damage, severe lung injury, or unconscious patients. Speak to your family and to your physicians regarding your healthcare wishes, should such an emergency situation arise. If no family is available to make such decisions on your behalf, and you have no previously documented instructions indicating how you would want the medical team to proceed with your care, a court-appointed legal healthcare proxy is typically appointed to make those decisions.

Q Have I made my decision about an organ donation?

Nobody plans to get in a car crash or become an innocent bystander of a shootout, but each of those people can save someone else's life with an organ donation.

Organ donation is possible once a patient has been declared brain dead. This can occur if a patient's brainstem, a part of the brain that controls the breathing and heart rate, is irreversibly damaged. At this point, the patient would be kept alive with the use of medications and artificial ventilation.

Many organs can be donated, such as the heart, kidneys, lungs, liver, bone marrow, blood, tendons, corneas, veins, heart valves and skin. Some of these organs can be transplanted up to 24 hours after a patient's heart has stopped beating. Organ donation gives the recipient a second chance at life and should be an open discussion among family members so that the proper decision can be made and the patient's wishes respected, if the scenario should arise.

Q Do I have a bleeding disorder surgeons need to be aware of?

A bleeding disorder, also known as, "coagulopathy," means that your blood does not clot properly and bleeding will take longer than normal to stop after any injury, including injury caused by surgery. Bleeding disorders can be inherited, such as Hemophilia or von Willebrand disease, or acquired (certain medications and some snakes' venom act as blood thinners). The importance of informing your medical team of any of these conditions or medications is that in the case of emergent surgery, appropriate planning in needed to ensure that you do not unexpectedly lose too much blood. Blood products and clotting factors can be prepared prior to surgery and given to any patient who needs them in order to prevent massive blood loss.

Q **Do I have any genetic abnormalities or rare medical conditions that emergency room physicians need to know about?**

Genetic abnormalities and rare medical conditions can alter the standard medical and surgical treatment in emergency surgery. Being rare, however, these conditions are not expected and you should inform your healthcare providers even if revealing such a condition may be embarrassing. These may be congenital conditions, like heart problems of childhood, kidney malformation, third nipples, and many other conditions.

It is also very important to discuss relatively rare conditions with your physicians to prevent unnecessary testing of what they think is an unexpected finding in a "standard" patient. Unexpected findings often raise the healthcare team's concerns and the possibility that such a finding is a result of a recent event, not a life-long condition, and are then investigated. Further investigation may be difficult for the patient to experience: physiologically, emotionally, and economically.

Q Am I allergic to any drugs? Should I be concerned about anaphylactic shock?

Allergic reactions are common and are caused by sensitivity to a particular substance, insect, animal or medication. An allergic reaction occurs when a patient's body and immune system are sensitized and respond excessively when exposed to this foreign material. At the extreme, the entire body reacts to the allergy within minutes in what is called, "anaphylactic shock," and patients typically have breathing difficulties, drops in blood pressure, lightheadedness or loss of consciousness, skin flushing and/or hives. If a known drug or latex allergy is present, it should be communicated to the medical team as alternatives for many medications exist. In the severe case of anaphylaxis, epinephrine is used to restore the blood pressure and maintain blood flow to the vital organs. Outside the hospital, epinephrine is available for sale from pharmacies in the form of an "EpiPen." Benadryl (Diphenhydramine) is given to stop the itching, swelling, and redness that often accompany an allergic reaction.

Q What does appendicitis look like and should I be concerned?

Patients with appendicitis usually experience pain in the abdomen, typically starting around the belly button and shifting toward the right lower portion. Emergency surgery is usually necessary.

Appendicitis is an inflammation of the appendix, a part of the intestines that can potentially rupture causing leakage into the body cavity. This is of grave concern and an emergency as the contents contain bacteria that can spread within your body leading to further complications and even death. The pain typically experienced begins near the belly button and later in the right lower quadrant of the abdomen. Nausea, vomiting, anorexia and fever are some signs and symptoms that are caused by appendicitis.

The treatment is an emergency appendectomy (surgical removal of the appendix). This procedure is commonly done laparoscopically (with special surgical cameras and tools), to leave the patient with minimal scarring (three or four small marks on the abdominal skin) and a much quicker recovery time. In some complicated cases of appendicitis, however, the abdomen has to be manually cut open in order to clear out the affected tissue.

Q I just experienced a traumatic injury. Should I inform the medical team if I have kidney disease?

Certain medical conditions affect the kidney. Some of the most common ones are diabetes, hypertension, and lupus. Certain medications such as aspirin, NSAIDS, metformin, lithium, and ACE Inhibitors are just a few medications that can cause damage to the kidneys. When a patient is seen in the trauma bay with a history of trauma to the head, abdomen, chest, or comes to the hospital with a broken bone, a common diagnostic tool is the CT scan. This machine uses complicated computerized mathematics and a series of x-rays to make a detailed image of the anatomy of the human body. In order to accurately and correctly visualize specific structures, however, physicians inject the patient with contrast dye to identify bleeding, damaged vessels, and/or specific organ injury. This contrast dye can potentially harm the kidneys, especially in those patients with poor kidney function due to congenital or chronic kidney disease. In these cases, make sure to tell your physicians if you have kidney problems so alternative imaging techniques that do not damage the kidneys can be employed.

Q Do I need to tell my doctors if I have any piercings or metallic implants?

In situations of trauma to the human body, a typical response is the inflammation and edema, which causes swelling of body tissues. The primary concern is that a piercing in the region of swelling can become extremely difficult to remove and may even squeeze and compromise the blood flow to a certain region of the body. The common example is a tight-fitting ring on a broken finger cutting off blood supply to the part of the finger beyond the ring. If this blood flow is not restored, death of the tissues beyond the piercing or ring will occur. Typical signs and symptoms experienced are pain, numbness, tingling, cold, lightening of the skin tone, paralysis, loss of blood pulses and a tense region of swelling.

Another concern about piercings, jewelry, or metal implants is in the cases when an MRI is necessary. This type of imaging modality uses a high power magnet that can move or displace certain metals as well as increase the temperature of implants and cause burns. Piercings can literally be ripped out of the skin by the MRI's magnets and metal implants like fake hips or knees can become extremely hot, causing pain and tissue damage if an MRI is performed. Any piercings or metallic implants should be reported to your medical team as soon as possible to prevent drastic complications that could lead to prolonging your medical treatment or damage to your body.

INTERNAL & PERIOPERATIVE MEDICINE

// See Disclaimer on page 1 of this book before reading this chapter.

Authors:

FREDERICK MA, MS-IV
St. George's University School of Medicine

Editors:

GEORGE GANDEV, M.D.
Attending Physician, Pulmonary Medicine & Critical Care
Lutheran Medical Center, Brooklyn, NY

MICHAEL BROUKHIM, M.D.
Cardiology Fellow, Urban Community Cardiology Fellowship Training Program
Mount Sinai Medical Center, NY, NY

Q I always have my blood drawn, and my last blood work was fine 6 months ago. Why is it that I need my blood drawn again before this surgery?

It is important practice for physicians and surgeons to order routine preoperative screening tests and blood tests on all patients, whom may be otherwise be asymptomatic or "as well as they can be." Large populations of patients may have common medical conditions including diabetes, hypertension, liver disease, kidney disease, or heart disease. Although the surgery that patients receive may not seem related or linked to their medical conditions, blood tests provide valuable information on a patient's baseline and general health status. This will allow for better assessment of the patient and also optimize their surgical success rates. Depending on the type and intensity of the surgery, the patient may be given a lot of fluids, certain antibiotics, and medications that can affect his or her general state of health.

So what types of information do doctors get from the vials of blood taken from me?

One vial is called a "Complete blood count" (CBC). This measures the amount of red blood cells, white blood cells, and hemoglobin in our blood. This is important to know as patients with 'anemia' or low hemoglobin may not be fit enough for surgery or may require a blood transfusion to keep them safe. This is also very relevant for patients with a history of blood loss, whether acute or chronic. The CBC also offers information on the patient's white blood count, which may help doctors make decisions about the patient's immune system function before and after surgery. Platelets are cells that help blood coagulate and form a clot. This may be very relevant for patients with a history of bruising or bleeding!

Another vial provides information about patient electrolytes – the ions and electrically conductive substances that make Gatorade rich! Electrolytes provide physicians with a wealth of information about the patient, including insight into the patient's kidney function, medication use, and heart function. Abnormal electrolytes, like low potassium, require correction to avoid a potentially dangerous situation!

Coagulation factors, prothrombin time and partial thromboplastin time, are clotting factors that need to be known by physicians if there is a risk of bleeding. Abnormalities in coagulation factors may be due to medications (most frequently Coumadin (warfarin), Heparin, or antibiotics), liver disease, malnutrition, or hereditary bleeding disorders.

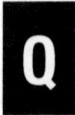

Q I am (or, my wife is) pregnant and may require surgery. Is there anything I need to know? Are there any risks involved?

In general, all elective non-obstetric surgeries are avoided due to unnecessary additional risks placed on the unborn child. With advancement in clinical imaging, such as high-resolution ultrasound, MRI, and other diagnostic tools, physicians are able to reduce and delay the need for surgery. However, there are general emergent conditions that have clear indications for surgery for pregnant patients. The most commonly occurring surgeries for pregnant women are acute appendicitis, acute cholecystitis (gall bladder inflammation), trauma, and gynecological diseases or cancers. Potential concerns for surgery and anesthesia for pregnant patients include miscarriage, bleeding, infections, and teratogenic (birth defect-causing) effects that may harm the fetus. Benefits and risks vary depending on both the pregnant patient's health status and the type of surgery; therefore, it is important to ask your physician or surgeon about the specific benefits and risks of your surgery.

Q I am having a surgery not related with the heart. Why does my pre-existing heart condition matter?

It is important for patients with pre-existing heart conditions to have a thorough heart risk assessment because it can influence the outcome of the surgery and the effects of anesthesia. With a good understanding of the patient's heart function, serious complications such as heart attacks and organ damage can be avoided. Statistically speaking, patients with a previous heart attack undergoing surgery have a risk of having a heart attack after surgery of approximately three percent. Patients diagnosed with peripheral vascular disease have a less than one percent chance of having a heart attack after non-cardiac surgery.

So what heart and cardiovascular conditions should be investigated?

Chest pain upon exertion, also known as angina, congestive heart failure, previous heart attacks, heart valve irregularities or replacement, previous heart surgery, peripheral vascular diseases, heart murmurs, or bruits in the neck.

What symptoms should you let your doctor know about that may be related to the heart?

If you feel chest pain or discomfort after walking, short of breath after walking, palpitations or feeling as if your heart is beating irregularly or fast, recent worsening in energy and ability to perform regular activities, jaw or neck pain after walking, or arm discomfort after walking.

Some classic diagnostic tests typically performed include chest x-ray, electrocardiogram (ECG or EKG), and echocardiograms, which provide a general assessment of the heart. However further testing may be required at times, depending on both the individual patient and the type of surgery.

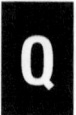

Q **I am not taking any new medications but I do take some long term medications. Does my physician/surgeon have to know about this?**

When patients are evaluated or scheduled for a surgery, it is important that patients also report what medications one is taking as it may affect the outcome and success of the surgery. In the operation, patients may be exposed to different types of anesthetics, pain medications, and will be experiencing varying degrees of bleeding depending on the nature of the operation.

Furthermore, after surgery patients will need some recovery time to regain strength and help wound healing. Medications that are especially important and may require modification in dosage includes blood pressure medications and diabetes medications. Blood thinning medications such as Aspirin, Plavix, Warfarin, and Heparin often require discontinuation as they may increase the risk of bleeding during and after surgery. Typically, Warfarin should be discontinued anywhere between five to seven days prior to surgery. Although you should tell your surgeon about all your medications, some of the following are particularly important medications to mention to your physician: selective estrogen modulators (SERMS), antidepressants, immune modifying drugs or cancer chemotherapy, and medications for thyroid disease.

Q I take herbal supplements. Are they considered to be medication?

Herbal supplements, medicinal teas, and plant-products are common nutritional supplements that many people take, whether they may be for health or cultural reasons. Although these products are natural, they may not always be safe for the body and may have some impact on surgery. There are very few published research articles at the moment for herbal supplements as they relate to surgery. However, the American Society of Anesthesiologists (ASA) has recommended stopping all herbal supplements 2-3 weeks before any operation. In relation to heart surgery, a study found that using herbal preparations can have negative side effects on the outcome and success of surgery. It was found that Echinacea, Ephedra, Gingko biloba, Garlic, Ginseng, St. John's Wort, Valerian root, and Kava created complications including low blood sugar, cardiovascular instability, drug interaction with anesthetic agents during surgery, and the potential to increase bleeding. Herbal supplements' ability to modify our liver metabolism, blood viscosity, and change our blood flow dynamics is the reason why some of these compounds can be dangerous in untested waters (the operating room).

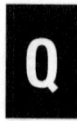 **I am going for surgery. What can I do to enhance my recovery time and healing process after the operation? Is bed rest a good idea?**

After the operation, patients need to recuperate and allow for normal wound healing, which can take up to two weeks. Patients undergoing musculoskeletal operations also require physiotherapy, which can take months for full range of motion and natural function to return. Immediately after surgery, patients will need to rest and recover from the anesthetics.

Patients should communicate well with the medical staff, including the physicians and nurses on how they want their pain managed and report how much pain they may be experiencing. Everyone has a different level of pain tolerance, fear or anxiety of pain, and cultural interpretation of pain. Patients need to understand that pain can be managed better if they communicate their feelings of discomfort. Good pain management can improve outcomes of major operations.

Furthermore, patients will have dressings over their incisions and possible drainage tubes. The outer layer of skin typically closes within 48 hours after an operation, but the inner layers may take longer to regain normal strength. It is important to allow time for full recovery of the incision sites.

Patients may ask for the type of stitching they may prefer in certain operations. Some stitches may dissolve while others are removed after a period of time. If they have to be removed, the patient will need to be seen shortly after surgery.

Although bed rest was once the gold standard to patient recovery, it is important for patients to start mobilizing when possible. Although pain may arise upon movement, it is encouraged that patients mobilize as tolerated. This prevents complications such as deep vein thrombosis, which is caused by lack of blood movement and clotting in the veins. A serious consequence to this condition is blood clots going to the lungs!

Q

I have had surgery as an outpatient recently and I am experiencing a fever right now. Does this mean I have an infection?

With the introduction of minimally invasive surgeries, there has been a surge in the number of outpatient surgical procedures in North America. Patients may develop a fever within a day. In most cases, this is due to a non-infectious process called atelectasis, which is caused by collapses of the lung's microscopic airways. This often happens after an operation because of both decreased strength for breathing due to pain or tight bandages, and excessive use of painkillers, which may suppress patients' breathing. Patients can avoid lying flat and lie down at a 45-degree angle to improve their breathing. Patients are also encouraged to use a device called an incentive spirometer, which can help expand the lungs and minimize atelectasis – this tool can be found at any hospital.

Although atelectasis is a common cause for fever on the first day, there are other causes that may include pneumonia, incisional site infections, urinary tract infections, or other less common infections. If patients experience other symptoms in addition to fever, including chest pains, excessive sweating, and/or shortness of breath, patients should contact their physician or call 911. Surgical site infections are very unlikely to occur during the first few days. A wound infection may present as a very tender, hot, and red area with or without pus. This symptom should be promptly examined by a physician, as the patient may require treatment. If a patient receives a urinary catheter (drainage tube), the patient will need to keep an eye on any urinary discomfort or symptoms that may contribute to the fever.

ANESTHESIOLOGY & PAIN MANAGEMENT

// See Disclaimer on page 1 of this book before reading this chapter.

Authors:

OGNJEN "OGI" VISNJEVAC, MS-IV
St. George's University School of Medicine

Editors:

LANCE W. WAGNER, M.D.
Clinical Assistant Professor, Anesthesiology
SUNY Downstate School of Medicine
SUNY Downstate Medical Center, Brooklyn, NY
Chairman, Department of Anesthesiology
Lutheran Medical Center, Brooklyn, NY

Q **Should I have a discussion with my anesthesiologist before surgery? What kinds of questions should I ask? What is the anesthesiologist's job, anyway?**

The anesthesiologist is in charge of much more than putting each patient to sleep. Generally speaking, the anesthesiologist's job is (1) to ensure patient safety and (2) to make the operative experience as comfortable and painless as possible. Specifically, he or she will look at your blood work, x-rays, and ECG results to make sure it is reasonably safe for you to undergo surgery. Additionally he or she will discuss your past medical and surgical history with you before surgery, looking out for things like a history of panic attacks, asthma, snoring, chest pains not related to activity, medication for anxiety, excessive alcohol intake or binge drinking, use of herbal supplements, a history of serious reaction to anesthesia by you or a family member (blood relative), a history of having a drug allergy, and/or a sensitivity to latex. Each of these things, and others not mentioned in the list, may suggest an increased risk for you to undergo anesthesia for your surgery and should be discussed with the anesthesiologist to ensure your safety. The anesthesiologist will care for your medical conditions during your surgery.

Remember that the anesthesiologist's job is to keep you safe, so it is very important to tell them your entire medical history. Do not leave anything out because disclosing a complete past medical and surgical history can often reveal very important information that could prevent heart attacks, strokes, and other serious complications. If you are concerned about something in your past medical or surgical history, or are worried about a specific complication of your surgery, you should discuss these concerns with the anesthesiologists, surgeon, and any other medical professional involved in your care.

In addition to focusing on your safety, the anesthesiologist will administer medications that produce anesthesia (a state of unconsciousness without sensation) and analgesia (no pain), along with medications that act on each patient's vital signs (heart rate, blood pressure, temperature, respiratory rate) to meet the desired effects needed for your surgery. If you have any questions regarding the medications to be used for your surgery, do no hesitate to ask the anesthesiologist.

The anesthesiologist will be monitoring your body functions with advanced electronic monitors to help insure your safety. The anesthesiologist will also make sure that the effects of these medications are adequately reversed for you to go to the recovery room, and then on to your hospital bed or to your home.

Lastly, the anesthesiologist is the person who is in charge of resuscitating a patient in the rare case that something goes wrong during the operation. Fortunately, such emergency situations are not common and, if they do occur, hospital staff are trained for emergency procedures and will not hesitate to lend a helping hand. If you have any concerns regarding resuscitation, or wish not to be resuscitated if something goes wrong, please discuss this with your anesthesiologist, surgeon, and everyone else involved in your medical care.

Q Why can't I eat before surgery?

Generally, surgeons and anesthesiologists will ask you not to eat or drink anything after midnight, the night before your surgery because there is a risk that, while under anesthesia, you will vomit what you ate. Vomiting on its own is an undesired effect and may not seem so serious, but patients who are under anesthesia can also inhale their stomach contents (a process called "aspiration"). Under normal day-to-day conditions, most people have a reflex at the back of the throat that causes the epiglottis, a floppy lid-like structure that sits above the trachea (AKA windpipe) to reflexively protect the airways by acting as a lid at the top of the trachea. This reflex happens every time something touches the back of the throat, whether due to swallowing or vomiting, and it is the reason why most people do not accidently start choking from inhaled chunks of food with every meal we eat.

Under anesthesia, however, this reflex is very often suppressed, meaning that the epiglottis will not close over the windpipe if vomit comes up from the stomach and into the throat. Hence, it is likely that vomit and stomach contents would end up in the lungs, a very dangerous scenario where stomach acid and undigested food in the lungs can lead to structural lung damage and pneumonia, and sometimes death. Often patients will be given a special antacid medication to help avoid this complication as well.

There are some procedures, like colonoscopies, bariatric surgery, colon resection or any other bowel surgery, in which an additional step is taken to empty one's bowels. Patients are given medications to take to induce diarrhea in an attempt to clean out the bowels before the procedure. This is beneficial because it provides surgeons with a good view of the intestines, not obscured by feces, and if the bowel is perforated or cut during the surgery, there will be less chance of infection if feces are not present to spill throughout the exposed abdomen. Such a spill causes infection along with a rather painful and potentially life-threatening condition called, "peritonitis," – inflammation of the inner abdominal wall.

Q **Should I continue taking my home-medications right up until the time of my surgery?**

This is, again, a very individual-dependent question and each medication should be addressed on its own. This issue is best discussed with your personal doctor, but you should also discuss it with your surgeon and anesthesiologist.

In most cases, people continue taking their medications right up until the day of surgery, but doctors will often require you to stop taking certain medications, like blood thinners for example, if they believe your risk of blood loss during surgery outweighs the risk of not taking that medication. Again, such risks are evaluated on an individual basis and must be discussed with your personal doctor, your surgeon, and your anesthesiologist.

Q I saw the movie "Awake." What if I wake up during my surgery?

Firstly it is important to note that not all surgeries require the patient to be asleep, and in some it is very beneficial to the medical team to get feedback from the patient regarding the progress of the surgery. Some patients may elect to be awake for their procedure while others may require deep sedation.

With mild to moderate sedation, this state of "awareness" can certainly be present. Under deeper sedation, such as general anesthesia, awareness is very rare. Some particular types of surgery, like heart surgery and emergency surgery, are associated with an increased incidence of patient awareness during surgery. Fortunately, this awareness phenomenon is not common. It is not yet definitively known whether some people become aware of their surgery because they metabolize the anesthetic medications faster than the average person, thereby needing higher doses of anesthetic to stay fully sedated, or whether there is another cause that predisposes certain people to become aware during surgery while the majority of others stay pleasantly asleep and pain-free.

Despite cases where the exact cause of awareness is not known, anesthesiologists are nonetheless able to treat the symptoms by monitoring each patient during surgery for signs of pain, discomfort, and awakening in order to adjust the medications required for that particular patient to stay safe and comfortable in the operating room.

In many cases, the state of awareness happens in response to complications during surgery and is a result of lowered amounts of anesthetic agents. For example, the anesthesiologist, whose job is primarily patient safety before patient comfort, may have to decrease the amount anesthetic the patient is receiving if the patient has significant blood loss, experiences problems breathing, or suffers from heart failure during the surgery. The anesthesiologist must balance patient comfort with medication side effects such as low blood pressure, depression of breathing, or prolonged unconsciousness.

Q I am getting a minor elective procedure. Do I need to be put under general anesthesia?

Although each patient's case is unique, the answer is often, "no, you don't need general anesthesia." Short or easy procedures like mole removal surgery or carpal tunnel repair often do not require general anesthesia and can be effectively treated by nerve block, sedation, pain medications, and/or local anesthetic. Other short and easy procedures like dilatation and curettage, a gynecological procedure, or colonoscopy, a gastrointestinal procedure, are not pleasant and patients usually prefer to be more deeply sedated for the duration of such procedures. Be aware that many of the medications used in sedation are the same as medications used during general anesthesia.

It will be important to discuss the anesthetic options of your case with your surgeon and your anesthesiologist, along with any other individual involved in your care. Keep in mind that the choice for which type of anesthesia should be a happy compromise between patient safety and patient comfort.

Q **I am getting major surgery. Can I stay awake?**

This depends on your state of health and the risks involved in the particular surgery. Procedures like knee replacements are major surgeries, but can be done with spinal or epidural anesthesia and do not require you to be unconscious for the operation. Some hernia repairs can be done with conscious sedation and a combination of local and intravenous (IV) pain medications. Abdominal or chest surgery typically requires general anesthesia. Again, in trying to decide the best mode(s) of anesthesia for each patient, the focus will be patient safety and patient comfort. Everyone wants the patient to come out of the OR safe, pain free, and in a better state than they came in, so discuss your goals for anesthesia (like staying awake) with your anesthesiologist and your surgeon in order to see if such goals would be possible, given the risks associated with your particular surgery.

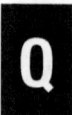 **I have a family member that had a bad reaction to anesthesia. What does that mean for me?**

There are rare cases that people cannot metabolize some of the anesthetic medications used for anesthesia because of a genetic mutation that does not allow them to break down those specific medications. An example of such a condition is called "malignant hyperthermia." If you or anybody in your family has had a bad reaction to anesthesia, it is extremely important that you tell your anesthesiologist before the surgery begins because such problems are often caused by a genetic mutation that is present in multiple family members. The anesthesiologist can use alternate medications that are broken down by a different mechanism in a different part of the body in order to keep you safe.

Q | **I don't want to feel pain. What types of pain control are available?**

Every patient is unique and every procedure comes with a different type and amount of pain. Thus, each patient should discuss his or her requirement for pain control with their surgeon(s) and anesthesiologist(s).

There are many ways to control one's pain, including nerve blocks, numbing creams, and medication that can be taken by mouth, intravenously, or intramuscularly. Sometimes, better pain control is achieved by nerve blocks or epidural catheter placement. In minor procedures like removal of small skin lesions or lipomas, local anesthetic might be sufficient. This type of medication acts right at the site of incision, blocking the pain signal from ever being formed so that the sensation of pain is never felt by the brain. Other medications, administered by nerve block or epidural catheter, dull the transmission of the pain signal as it travels through those nerves to the brain, again preventing the sensation of pain from registering in the brain. Lastly, there are those medications that act directly on the brain so that the patient does not feel pain. Tylenol (acetaminophen) is the perfect example of such a centrally acting pain relief medication that acts on the brain directly to stop the feeling of pain.

Of course, if you have had allergic reaction to pain medications in the past or if you know you cannot take a certain pain medication for whatever reason, please let your anesthesiologist(s), surgeon(s), nurses, and other medical staff know. Likewise, it will be important to tell them if you have liver or kidney disease because pain medications are typically metabolized by either the liver or the kidney, or both, and damage to either organ may dictate that a different medication may need to be used for safer and more effective pain control. Lastly, if you have been taking pain relief medication on a regular basis, it will be important to let the anesthesiologist know that names of each of your pain relief medications, including over-the-counter medications, as well as the dosages of each mediation.

Q The "scary" question: What is the chance I will not wake up from my surgery?

Overall, the chances are extremely low that you will not wake from your surgery. Of course, this is not a question that can be simply explained or broadly applied because a lot of factors play into the individual risks of surgery. Your age, sex, state of health, past medical and surgical histories, the risks involved in this particular surgery, and your own personal reaction to anesthesia are just some of the variables that play in what is termed the, "preoperative" risk assessment." Since this assessment is entirely unique to the combination of you and your surgery, you should discuss it with your physicians to find out your own personal risk.

In general, however, there are some surgeries, like heart surgery, brain surgery, or traumatic emergency surgery (examples: gunshot wounds, stab wounds, motor vehicle accidents) that carry greater risk. If your past medical histories include heart disease, kidney problems, a history of previous heart attack(s), stroke(s), recurrent infections, asthma or chronic lung disease, or other health problems, make sure to tell both your anesthesiologist and the rest of your medical team because these factors increase the risks of you undergoing all types of surgery.

In addition, you may also want to compare the risks of getting surgery with the risks of not getting surgery, keeping in mind the expected quality of life you would be living with in each scenario.

Q I don't want to get addicted to pain medications. Should I ask for medicines to treat my pain?

This is a very common concern. Pain management is extremely important and is taken very seriously, but some pain medications can be abused to cause addiction. You should know that you have the right to refuse pain relieving medications or procedures, like nerve blocks, just the same as you have the right to refuse anything that is to be done to you, but you can also discuss your concerns regarding addiction to pain medication with the hospital staff to find a solution that is personally tailored to you, your goals, your surgery, and your pain control needs. There are medical specialists who deal with acute and/or chronic pain on a regular basis and you might need to discuss your concerns and wishes with them in situations where a lot of pain is expected as a result of your condition or your surgery.

GENERAL SURGERY

// See Disclaimer on page 1 of this book before reading this chapter.

Authors:

BORIS SRVANTSTIAN, MS-IV
St. George's University School of Medicine

Editors:

OSAMA ELSAWY, D.O.
Chief Resident, General Surgery Residency Program
Lutheran Medical Center, Brooklyn, NY

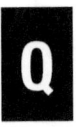

Q **I have gallstones. Do I need surgery? If so, what type of surgery do I need? What are the possible complications?**

The need for surgery depends on several factors, primarily the presence or absence of symptoms. In asymptomatic patients, surgery is not recommended unless the patient is immunocompromised, has a porcelain (calcified) gallbladder, and/ or gallstones that are larger than 3 cm, because these findings are associated with a higher chance of developing gallbladder cancer. If the patient has symptoms of gallstone disease, then surgery is recommended. The most common surgery is called laparoscopic cholecystectomy. This is a minimally invasive surgery with very small scars, usually less than half an inch in length. Due to the gallbladder's proximity to the liver and its structures, a possible (although highly rare) complication may be serious liver damage.

Q I have acid reflux (AKA GERD or gastro-esophageal-reflux disease) and the medications are not helping. Can surgery help me?

GERD is not fun to have and it makes its presence known with an achy or sharp pain in the chest that many may confuse for a heart attack. The underlying cause of this disease is the weakness of the sphincter (muscular ring that acts as a valve) that connects the esophagus and the stomach. This weakness allows some of the acid from the stomach to reflux back into the esophagus after a meal and move upwards towards the throat. This is more common when the patient is laying flat. Initial therapy is with medications such as proton pump inhibitors that will lower the production of acid, as well as lifestyle modifications such as losing weight and not eating before bedtime. However, there are cases where these approaches do not work and surgery is needed. Every patient needs preoperative evaluation which involves visualizing the esophagus with a camera and performing a biopsy (to make sure that no malignancy is present) and esophageal manometry which helps measure the pressures inside the esophagus during swallowing to make sure that the patient is able to normally swallow food after the surgery. The operation is called Nissen fundoplication and it involves taking part of the stomach and wrapping it around the lower esophageal sphincter to give it more tone in order to prevent reflux.

Q | I have an inguinal hernia. What is it? What are my surgical options?

An inguinal hernia is the protrusion of the abdominal contents through an opening in the groin area. There are two types, direct and indirect inguinal hernias. The difference lies in the anatomic relation of the herniated intestine to the inferior epigastric vessels. The repair for both types is identical. This is an elective surgery, which means that the patient can choose to avoid surgery and live with the hernia, but this means that the patient will not be able to lift any heavy objects and any increase in the abdominal pressure such as defecating, laughing or sneezing will cause the hernia to slide in and out and cause some amount of pain.

Furthermore, the patient always runs the risk of having the hernia become incarcerated (get stuck in the opening), which means that the blood supply to that part of the bowel will be cut off and the bowel may die. This is a surgical emergency. There are several surgical options that are available to the patient. The patient can either opt for an open repair, which typically leaves a 3- to 6-inch long scar, or a laparoscopic repair, which leaves smaller scars. The goal of all of these repairs is to put the abdominal contents back into the abdomen and close the defect through which the bowel herniated. The procedure technique mostly depends on the surgeon's preference and the cost to the patient. The most common complications that may arise from this procedure are damage to the nearby nerves and wound infection. These complications occur anywhere from 1%-10% of the time. After a successful surgery, the patient is usually advised not to lift anything heavy for the first 6 weeks after which a gradual progress to normal lifting may occur.

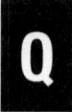

Q **I was treated for a spontaneous pneumothorax, and my doctor told me that it was because of the "apical blebs" that she saw on my imaging study. What is a spontaneous pneumothorax? What are apical blebs? Can it happen again? How do I avoid it?**

Spontaneous pneumothorax is a common condition in young healthy patients. It is called spontaneous because there was no external trauma, penetrating wound, or other event that caused the damage. Most common reason for this condition is the rupture of what are called, "apical blebs." These blebs are thin-walled bubble-like structures found on the edges of the lungs. They are formed due to internal lung defects and may spontaneously rupture or rupture during intense exercise. This leads to air escaping into the space between the lungs and the chest wall, which will cause an elevation in the pressure. This pressure will soon exceed the pressure inside the lungs, and cause the damaged lung to collapse. The patient will have sudden difficulty in breathing and sharp chest pain during the rupture. This requires immediate treatment in an emergency department, usually with placement of a chest tube. This helps re-expand the damaged lung and allows the patient to breath again. However, if this condition continues to occur, the best mode of treatment would be the surgical removal of these blebs followed by a procedure called pleurodesis (irritating the lining of the lungs to make them thicker in order to avoid a future pneumothorax).

Q Does everyone have to have a Foley catheter inserted for his or her surgery?

A Foley catheter is a thin sterile tube inserted into the bladder to drain urine through the urethra. It is used to empty the bladder at the start of almost every surgery requiring general anesthesia or other forms of sedation and is typically removed as soon as it is no longer needed. For long surgeries, it is typically left in place to monitor urine production (which reflects the state of a patient's hydration and kidney function) during most operations performed under general or spinal anesthesia that last more than an hour.

In urology (and gynecology), the Foley catheter is typically removed after draining the bladder at the start of the procedure if the urologist (or gynecologist) uses tools that are inserted through the urethra.

Foley catheters may be used in other, non-surgical, scenarios as well, especially when a patient is having difficulty urinating. This may be a short-term solution, lasting only a few hours or days. Alternately, a catheter with a bag may be placed for the patient to use long-term at home if that patient cannot be treated in other, more comfortable, ways.

Q | I have liver cirrhosis. Can surgery help me?

"Liver cirrhosis" is severe damage to the structure of the liver, an organ responsible for detoxifying our blood and making hundreds of helpful chemicals to keep us healthy. The most common causes of liver cirrhosis are excessive alcohol intake and hepatitis B or C infection. Two consequences of liver cirrhosis are (1) "portal hypertension," a concept describing the disruption of normal blood flow in the abdomen, and (2) decreased overall liver function, which means prolonged bleeding, metabolic dysfunction, and weakening of the immune system.

Patients often first show signs of portal hypertension by vomiting or coughing up blood coming from a burst vein in their stomach or esophagus. These veins get distended and burst because of the disruption of normal blood flow caused by liver cirrhosis. At the same time, patients may have a distended fluid-filled abdomen (called "ascites"), swollen legs or an enlarged spleen.

Because the liver makes clotting factors and releases a compound called, "thrombopoitin," which increases the production of special clotting cells, called platelets, it is vital in the body's day-to-day ability to stop any bleeding. Liver cirrhosis (severe damage to the liver), therefore leads to bleeding problems.

The portal hypertension is the most serious complication of the disease because it may cause the rupture of these dilated vessels and lead to excessive blood loss which may cause death. At first, medications will be tried, but if this approach does not work, the best next step is a surgical procedure called Transjugular Intrahepatic Portal-Systemic Shunt (TIPS). This procedure is relatively safe and quick and it provides great relief because it lowers the portal pressure in the veins that caused the excessive spontaneous bleeding.

Unfortunately, even after this surgical procedure, the function of the liver is still compromised and the patient will be at risk of developing neurological problems (called, "hepatic encephalopathy"). In such cases, treatment for this complication of TIPS is to put the patient on medication called lactulose and to limit the protein intake in the diet. This surgical procedure does not cure the patient, it only relives the symptoms. The only definitive cure for liver cirrhosis is liver transplantation but that, too, has its own complications.

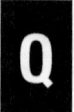

Q I have Crohn's disease, and my doctor told me that I could end up with a small bowel obstruction. How will I know if I get it? What should I do if I get these symptoms? How would I be treated?

Crohn's disease is an inflammatory type of disease that may involve any part of the digestive system from the mouth to the anus. The most common area that it involves is the small intestines. One of the features of Crohn's disease is to cause the narrowing of some parts of the small bowel called "strictures." These strictures are responsible for the small bowel obstruction that may occur in many patients with this disease. Some signs that a patient may have an obstruction include nausea and vomiting, cramps, abdominal pain, abdominal distention, no bowel movements, and if it is a complete obstruction, no passage of gas. If these symptoms persist, the best thing to do for the patient is to go to the emergency room and get immediate treatment. Any delay in treatment puts the patient at serious complications of bowel wall rupture. The initial management of small bowel obstruction will be the placement of a Nasogastric Tube (NG), which is a small tube with perforations that is inserted either through the mouth or the nose all the way into the stomach and hooked up to a vacuum in the room. This is an uncomfortable procedure and most patients don't like it, but it is necessary because it helps to reduce the distention by sucking the gas and fluid out. This will be followed by the standard procedure of placing the patient on TPN (total paranteral nutrition), which means the patient will be artificially fed through the vein, and an intravenous (IV) line will be placed for adequate hydration. All of this is done to allow the bowel to rest and try to clear the obstruction. If the obstruction still persists with this non surgical management, then surgical intervention is needed.

There are two approaches that can be taken, depending on the number of strictures. If there is only one stricture present, then it is removed from the small intestine and the healthy parts are reconnected to each other. If there are multiple strictures, cutting them out runs the risk of removing too much bowel, which would leave the patient with a new set of problems. Instead a Stricturoplasty is performed which is essentially a procedure that just dilates the stricture without removing it.

The patient should also be aware that some problems may arise after this procedure. The most common place that is affected by Crohn's disease is the terminal ileum (the junction between the small bowel and the large bowel); its removal will precipitate some digestive and blood-related problems. The terminal ileum is responsible for absorbing bile acids and Vitamin B12, a vitamin required for the formation of red blood cells. Thus, patients who have this procedures should take vitamin B12 intramuscular injections to avoid becoming anemic (having low amounts of red blood cells). The bile acids help in the digestion of fats, thus the patient may experience diarrhea, weight loss, and difficulty absorbing some essential vitamins, (ADEK) which will also need to be replaced in addition to Vitamin B12.

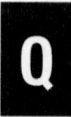

Q **I've been diagnosed with an abdominal aortic aneurysm (aka AAA or "triple-A"). What does that mean for me? Do I need surgery? Is there anything I can do to avoid surgery? How often should I go see a doctor?**

The most important aspect of having a diagnosis of abdominal aortic aneurysm (AAA) are adequate follow-ups with a physician, using regular abdominal ultrasounds to monitor for any change in size of the aneurysm. On average, the diameter of the AAA enlarges about 4mm/year. Once it reaches 5 cm in diameter, surgical intervention is recommended because it is prone to spontaneous rupture, which will lead to large amount of blood loss, shock, and sometimes death. More than 50% of patients die on the way to the hospital when an AAA ruptures. Thus the only way to avoid surgery is if the aneurysm does not enlarge, or the patient is not a good surgical candidate due to other health problems.

The procedure itself is pretty straightforward. The surgeon makes an incision in the abdomen, locates the aorta, cuts of the blood flow to the area that is needed for the surgery by using clamps, opens the aorta, cleans out the plaque (which most likely caused this condition), and places a graft inside the aorta so that it holds its normal shape. The most common complication of this surgery is something called "third spacing." This means that the water in your body is not in the veins, but is somewhere else, such as the lungs or the abdomen. After about 3 days or so spent in the hospital to monitor the patient during the initial phases of recovery, the body hopefully gets rid of the extra fluid. Some other complications may be impotence in males, due to the damage to the nerves that pass over the aorta and supply the groin area. For this, the patient should see an urologist (a specialist of the urinary tract and groin) for a more complete evaluation.

Other, more serious complications, include dead bowel (mostly involves a part of the colon) due to the surgical procedure when the surgeon was clamping the vessels to stop the blood flow. Most of the time this happens because the patient had bad secondary blood flow to the bowel due to plaque build up in other blood vessels that were supposed to supply the bowel while the surgery was happening. If the bowel has completely died, than another surgery will be needed to cut that part of the colon out. If it is only partially dead, the surgeon will admit the patient to the hospital for close observation to see if the bowel recovers from the injury. Finally, the most serious complication is the failure of the graft itself. Most often this results from contamination by bacteria that are present on the skin, which somehow find their way to the graft. The treatment involves the complete removal of the graft and performing a bypass surgery (like heart bypass, only with the aorta).

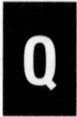

Q **I found out that I have colon cancer and I need surgery. Will the surgery cure me? Are there any complications I should watch out for?**

Colon cancer is a highly malignant cancer and the cure depends on whether the cancer spread to other parts of the body. Hence part of the pre-operative work up includes chest X-ray, blood tests for tumor markers, and liver function tests. If the liver function test is not normal, a CT scan is warranted to see if there are any lesions present. These procedures will help the surgeon assess the spread of the cancer.

The patient should always discuss the postoperative risks of any surgery. With this type of surgery, risks such as wound infection, a possible leak from the site where the bowel was reconnected, and a potential urinary problem due to damage of the ureters are all possibilities. Before the surgery, the bowel will need to be prepped by giving the patient a laxative to "clean" the bowel. This will be followed by antibiotics to kill off the bacteria that inhabit our intestines and to prevent the risk of post operative wound infections. This is a serious surgery that involves a large amount of the bowel to be removed with other supporting structures in an attempt to make sure that the cancer will not come back.

If the entire cancer has been removed and there was no sign of spread, than the patient is considered cured, and is followed by the doctor to see if there is recurrence anywhere else in the body. If the cancer has spread before the surgery, however, a cure is unlikely and the surgery will be palliative in nature by providing the patient relief from the mass effect of the cancer in the bowel.

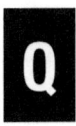 **Q** **My doctor told me I have diverticuli in my colon. What are diverticuli? Will I need surgery in the future?**

Diverticuli are small outpouchings in the large colon, most commonly present on the left side. The most common cause of diverticuli is inadequate dietary fiber, leading to increased strain on the large intestine and elevated pressure inside the bowel, causing small parts of the large bowel to herniate through natural weakness in the bowel wall. These diverticuli will eventually cause bleeding because they will erode through nearby small blood vessels. Luckily, most diverticular bleeds stop spontaneously, but there is a 25% chance that these diverticuli will re-bleed and a 20% chance that surgery will be necessary. In cases when diverticuli bleed continuously or excessively, there is great risk that the patient will end up in hemorrhagic shock. If untreated, this may cause death, thus, surgery becomes the treatment of choice.

Before the surgery, the surgeon will have to localize the site of the bleed. Once the source of the bleeding is located, the surgeon can proceed with either a right or left "hemicolectomy" (removal of the affected part of the colon). This will be followed by reconnecting the healthy bowel together. The reason that the surgeon takes out such a large portion of the colon, instead of just the localized area with the bleeding, is so that there is less chance of repeat bleeding.

CARDIOTHORACIC SURGERY: HEART, LUNGS, & ESOPHAGUS

// See Disclaimer on page 1 of this book before reading this chapter.

Authors:

OGNJEN "OGI" VISNJEVAC, MS-IV
St. George's University School of Medicine

Editors:

ADAM E. SALTMAN, M.D., PH.D.
Assistant Professor, Surgery
SUNY Downstate Medical Center, Brooklyn, NY

CHRISTOPHER J. VARUGHESE, M.D.
Fellow in Cardiovascular Medicine
Mount Sinai School of Medicine
Mount Sinai Hospital, NY, NY

// HEART SURGERY

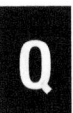 **Q** **Someone in my family had a heart attack recently. What treatment options are there?**

A "heart attack" is a very general term describing a blockage of one or more blood vessels supplying blood to the heart and often cause pressure-like chest pain, nausea, sweating, jaw and/or shoulder pain. Every heart attack is considered a medical emergency so **CALL 9-1-1 immediately** if you have any of the above symptoms! It is extremely important to treat heart attacks as soon as possible because damage to the heart muscle is often somewhat reversible. Treatment of heart attacks is a broad and expansive topic, but it can be simplified into (1) the initial treatment, (2) interventional and/or surgical procedures, and (3) long-term therapy.

The goals of the initial treatment of a heart attack are to restore blood flow to the heart and to determine both the cause of the heart attack and the amount of damage done to the heart muscle. In an ambulance and an emergency department, medications such as aspirin, nitroglycerine, beta-blockers, oxygen, and/or morphine are often administered to relieve some of the symptoms and slow the progression of heart muscle damage. An electrocardiogram ("ECG" or "EKG") is administered to help the medical team diagnose whether each patient's chest pain is caused by a heart attack and, if so, which area of the heart has been affected. If such measures are deemed appropriate by the medical team, the patient is taken to the cardiac catheterization laboratory (AKA "Cath Lab") to identify every blockage. This is often an essential step in the treatment of a heart attack because it will provide doctors with vital information necessary to administer effective treatment.

It is important to note that each and every patient's interventional and/ or surgical treatment plan will be unique, based upon a combination of their own medical and surgical histories, along with their current presentation, and the treatment capabilities of the medical facility they are in. If the medical facility is not equipped with a "Cath Lab", medications may be used to attempt to dissolve the clots that are causing the blockage. However, a facility equipped with a cardiac "Cath Lab" has the capability of opening the blocked vessel with a balloon, and placing a mesh cylinder or stent in the artery in an effort to keep that blood vessel open. Such decisions will vary based upon individual patient circumstances and, in some cases, such interventions will no longer be effective if too much time has passed between the onset of symptoms and the time of cardiac catheterization. Bypass surgery may be the best option in cases where other procedures are not likely to be effective or in cases where several vessels are significantly occluded at the same time. During this procedure, a healthy vessel (typically a vein from the leg or an artery from the chest wall) is used to shunt blood beyond the blockage to the area(s) of the heart starved of blood supply.

Long-term therapy is typically medical (managed by the personal medical doctor, internal medicine specialist, or cardiologist), not surgical, but there are situations when additional surgical procedures are recommended. Many people who have suffered through a heart attack develop irregular rhythms or arrhythmias of the heart, which are irregular electrical impulses and contractions of the heart muscle. These can be very dangerous and may even cause sudden death. If such complications cannot be controlled medically, a pacemaker or internal defibrillator may need to be placed. The pacemaker and the defibrillator are both small devices used to maintain the heart's rhythm (pacemaker) and shock the heart back to a normal rhythm (defibrillator) if it detects a life-threatening arrhythmia.

A heart attack is a very serious health problem and every individual case should be thoroughly discussed with the medical team to optimize the patient's short- and long-term care.

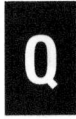

Q My cardiac catheterization showed that I have a decreased ejection fraction and "three – vessel disease." Do I really need bypass surgery? Are there any other options?

In recent years there has been much excitement and quite a bit of media attention on the advent and use of stents to treat clogged blood vessels in the heart. Stents act as cylinders that prop the vessel open and allow blood to travel downstream. Stents cannot, or should not, be used in certain circumstances.

The joint guidelines set out by the American College of Cardiologists and the American Heart Association (ACC-AHA) dictate that coronary artery bypass grafting (CABG), commonly referred to as "bypass surgery," is indicated in a specific subset of patients and has improved survival when compared to standard medical therapy. Coronary revascularization with CABG is thus recommended for patients with decreased left ventricular function, which is often diagnosed as a decreased ejection fraction, significant left main coronary artery disease, "3-vessel disease," and/or unstable angina.

It would be important to note that there are significant risks associated with CABG procedures and that the recovery process can be quite lengthy, but the above mentioned patients would be at even higher risk of morbidity and/or mortality when treated with conservative medical management.

Additionally, one should discuss co-morbid conditions, like lung or kidney disease, with the surgeon because these may affect the management recommendations, risks, and outcomes.

Q My doctor tells me I have a murmur. Does this mean I need surgery and, if so, how urgently do murmurs need to be treated? Do I need any special medical treatment just because I have a murmur?

Heart murmurs are "whoosh"-like sounds heard with a stethoscope. They are caused by turbulent blood flow through the heart valves. They can be innocent (not dangerous) or pathological (potentially dangerous).

Innocent murmurs are found most often in children and pregnant women. They do not need treatment because the heart is otherwise normal and no malfunction will develop. If your child has an innocent murmur, alert his or her doctor during regular check-ups so that it is noted in his or her medical records. If a murmur appears during pregnancy, this most likely reflects the extra maternal blood volume women have during pregnancy to support a growing fetus. A murmur associated with pregnancy will therefore resolve afterward.

Pathological heart murmurs may occur at any age, but usually appear in older adults. They always require treatment of some kind, as most will lead to heart failure eventually. Specific treatments are based upon the specific valve affected (aortic, mitral, etc.), and so each individual case should be discussed with one's personal medical doctor and a cardiologist or heart surgeon. In general, pathological murmurs increase the risk of infection on the valves (endocarditis), and therefore preventive antibiotics are needed for invasive procedures such as dental cleaning, colonoscopy, and others.

If you have a murmur, speak with your doctor(s) to see if you need treatment and, if so, what the recommended treatment is for your particular case.

Q **If I opt for heart surgery, will I be on medication afterward? For how long?**

Medication after heart surgery is prescribed for several reasons. There are treatments for pain control, constipation, anemia, water overload, blood pressure and heart function. Your doctors may also prescribe blood thinners, platelet-inhibitors, or rhythm-control drugs. Some of these are temporary and will be terminated after you recover (such as for pain and constipation), whereas others must be taken for life (such as aspirin, plavix, and/or beta-blockers). The duration and dosage of each medication will vary between patients and should be discussed with your doctors.

It is very important for you to review your current, past, and over-the-counter medication list with your physicians, because some medications will interact with the typical medications prescribed after heart-surgery and may have negative side effects.

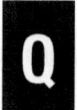

Q **How long is my expected recovery from open-heart surgery? When will I be able to resume normal activities? Drive a car? Return to work? Have sex? Be independent in activities of daily living?**

There are many factors to consider when discussing recovery from open-heart surgery so this issue should be discussed in detail on an individual basis with your surgeon. Typically, the first 5-7 days after the surgery will be spent in the hospital so that the hospital staff can observe and help with the recovery process and intervene if something goes wrong.

Initially, you will wake up from surgery in an intensive care unit with a nurse at your side. The first day or two is critical for managing your fluid balance, adjusting your medications, and removing any special tubes or intravenous lines.

Once most of these issues have resolved, you will be transferred to a regular patient floor to spend the rest of your stay. You will start to get out of bed. You will be eating your regular diet. A physical therapist will work with you as you start to recover your strength. More strenuous activities such as stair climbing will be undertaken with supervision, as you will be weak at first. After you have been walking by yourself and all of the medications are stabilized, you will be sent home. This is typically after 5 days or so.

Once out of the hospital, you will continue to recover for the next few months. Showering is permitted and encouraged, but bathing should be avoided for about one week. Driving is prohibited until you see your surgeon in follow-up, usually 3 – 6 weeks after surgery. Similarly, do not lift anything heavier than about 10 lbs or engage in sexual relations until you have seen your surgeon and discussed these activities with him.

Minimizing fatigue throughout the recovery process is very important. It is not uncommon to take frequent naps while you are recovering. If you feel tired, stop and rest. You will steadily build back your strength and endurance. Most patients are prescribed a period of cardiac rehabilitation after surgery exactly to help with healing and strength recovery.

During your recovery, always be alert for complications. Problems that require prompt medical attention are a fever of greater than 101.4° F (38° C); angina-like pain in your chest; swelling in your legs; oozing, pain, redness, or pus from the incisions (leg or chest); and clicking or instability at the chest incision. If you experience any of these, call your surgeon right away.

Full recovery time varies widely among patients. Some people feel well after only 3 or 4 weeks, whereas others may take 3 or 4 months to return to normal activities. Stay in touch with your surgeon so that he or she can monitor your progress. Of course, any troubling symptoms should be brought to the attention of the surgeon and/or personal medical doctor as soon as possible.

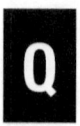 **My doctor saw a "coin lesion" on a routine chest x-ray. What is a coin lesion? Is this bad? Will I need surgery?**

A coin lesion is also called a "solitary pulmonary nodule". It is a circular mass that is surrounded by normal lung tissue. It is usually small, so most patients do not have any symptoms. Furthermore, it is almost impossible to tell the underlying cause of the coin lesion from the x-ray (infection, cancer, congenital lesion, lymph node, etc.). Therefore, further work up is required of all coin lesions.

The first step is to see if the coin lesion is new or if it was there on older x-rays. A new lesion would be more worrisome, and would typically prompt your doctor to obtain a computed tomograph (CT scan) of the chest. The CT scan yields much more information than a simple chest x-ray, both about the lesion and the lungs and other organs. A CT scan can also be used by an interventional radiologist to obtain a biopsy using a fine needle.

If a biopsy cannot be obtained using CT scan guidance, then a surgeon will typically be called to obtain one. Nowadays, lung biopsies can be obtained using minimally invasive techniques with cameras and thin instruments, such that the ribs do not need to be spread and no chest muscles need to be cut. Recovery from these video-assisted thoracic surgical (VATS) procedures is very quick, and most patients leave the hospital within 24 – 48 hours.

Q **I have been diagnosed with lung cancer. Is there any hope? Should I even bother with surgery? What about clinical trials?**

Whether or not you would need more extensive surgery than a VATS would depend upon many things. The first is whether or not it can be determined if you have cancer. If the biopsy is not conclusive, then it may be necessary to remove the entire lobe of the lung containing the lesion. If the biopsy did show cancer, however, then VATS can be used to sample lymph nodes in the chest and help stage the cancer. Early stage cancers typically would be treated by removing the entire lobe that contained the coin lesion. With later stage cancers, chemotherapy and radiation therapy would be used first and surgery used only after a good response has occurred.

Survival for early stage lung cancer is good, with 95% of patients living 5 years if a small lesion has been entirely removed and there are no signs of spread. Most patients do not even notice the small loss of lung function after surgery. Survival drops off quickly, however, if the lesion becomes larger, invades other structures or lymph nodes, or spreads outside the chest cavity. Early detection and removal remain the cornerstone of successful therapy. Once a cancer has been diagnosed, you should have a detailed discussion with your doctors about the stage of your cancer and the anticipated treatments, results, and alternatives available to you.

Clinical trials of experimental treatments may be an option for some patients with more advanced cancers, but the benefits and risks of each trial should be thoroughly discussed before enrolling. To look for a clinical trial that might be a good match, ask your physician or start by searching the following websites:

http://clinicaltrials.gov
Search: "Lung Cancer"

http://www.cancer.org/treatment/treatmentsandsideeffects/
clinicaltrials/app/clinical-trials-matching-service
(The official website of the American Cancer Society Clinical Trials Matching Service)

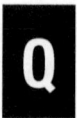

Q   My emphysema is no longer bearable. I can't breathe. Can surgery help me?

This is a complicated question with a controversial answer: Yes, sometimes.

Many cases of emphysema result from large bubbles ("bullae") forming in the lung. These bubbles do not participate in air exchange, and only serve to compress the "good" parts of the lung, making you short of breath. Theoretically, removing these bullae should allow the good parts of the lung to re-expand and participate in air exchange, making you feel better and breathe more easily. This operation is known as "lung volume reduction surgery" (LVRS). Unfortunately, the results of several large LVRS trials have been disappointing. Although most patients felt relief from their emphysema, they returned to a poor functional state after about two years. Therefore, the government stopped paying for these procedures and most surgeons have stopped performing them.

Another option is lung transplantation, where one or both lungs are removed entirely and replaced with one or two lungs taken from a deceased (cadaver) donor. Unfortunately, there are only about 1400 lung transplants every year in the United States, due to severe donor supply restrictions. Many more people need such transplants than there are organs available. Therefore, only severely ill patients who can be matched to a donor (same blood type, similar sized lungs) receive transplants. Of those who receive a donor lung, most enjoy a much better quality of life, but at the cost of taking many immunosuppressive drugs.

Because of these disappointing surgical results and the severe limitation of donor organs, new devices and procedures are being developed to help patients with severe emphysema. Most of the devices can be introduced into the lung using small cameras on flexible tubes (bronchoscopes) while the patient is awake and sedated. The patients can leave the hospital the same day. Currently they are in clinical trials (for example, see clinicaltrials.gov: trials NCT00207337, NCT00391612, NCT00730301, and NCT00475007); none are approved for sale in the US as of this writing.

Q I think my child inhaled something and is choking on it. What should I do?

If you think your child is choking, this is an emergency: Take him or her directly to the emergency room of the nearest hospital or call 911.

Children will put anything in their mouths and, if they do not swallow properly, objects like toys often get stuck in the airway. This blocks air from coming in and out of the lungs. It can be very distressing for the child and can be life-threatening. Do not delay seeking medical attention!

If the object can be seen at the back of the throat, it may be taken out without putting the child to sleep. If the object is too deep to be seen directly, however, its size and location can be identified by x-ray. It can then be taken out by using bronchoscopy, sometimes with a flexible tube and camera, other times with a rigid tube and grasping instruments. This is done with the child asleep.

If the object is successfully removed without any airway injuries, then a brief period of observation will be required. Your child can go home with you after that.

// ESOPHAGEAL SURGERY

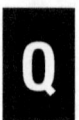 **I seem to be having problems swallowing. Do I need surgery?**

Although there are many esophageal conditions that can be treated medically, some problems of the esophagus are more serious and should be surgically corrected. Swallowing problems are often the first signs of some very concerning conditions such as cancer. They therefore should be promptly investigated. The most important thing is to tell your physician of your symptoms as soon as possible, so an early intervention can be done. Delaying serves no good purpose and may lead to a much less desirable result.

One of the first steps in investigating an esophageal problem is to look inside the esophagus with a camera on a flexible tube. This is called "esophagoscopy" and can be done while you are awake but sedated. It is an ambulatory procedure, so you can go home afterward. Pictures can be taken of any abnormalities, and samples (biopsies) can be sent to the pathologist for analysis. Complications are quite rare and the procedure is well tolerated by almost everyone.

Many benign problems such as strictures can even be treated through the esophagoscope. Balloons can be used to open the esophagus, for example, If acid-reflux changes are seen, then only medical treatment would usually be required.

If a cancer is diagnosed, then additional testing would be required to determine the stage of the cancer and what can be done about it: chemotherapy, radiation therapy, and/or surgery. These topics are very complex, so a detailed discussion among you and your physicians should take place once more diagnostic data is available. Fortunately, in this era much esophageal surgery can be done minimally invasively, allowing patients to leave the hospital and recover much faster while experiencing much less pain than ever before.

ORTHOPEDIC SURGERY: BONES, LIMBS, & MUSCLES

// See Disclaimer on page 1 of this book before reading this chapter.

Authors:

BORIS SRVANTSTIAN, MS-IV
St. George's University School of Medicine

Editors:

SHADI SHIHATA, M.D., FRCS(C)
Orthopedic Surgeon
University of Calgary
Foothills Medical Centre, Calgary, AB, Canada

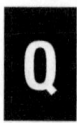

Q I have osteoarthritis in my knee(s). Will a total knee replacement improve my walking? Do I have any other options?

Osteoarthritis is a degenerative disease involving the cartilage of the weight bearing joints, which is most commonly caused by wear and tear throughout one's life. The knee joint is one of the most commonly affected joint, resulting in pain with every step, which is why this disease can be so debilitating. Normally, cartilage serves as a buffer between the two hard ends of the bones in the knee joint. Once this buffer is gone, however, the bones rub against each other and produce pain that can be anything from achy to excruciating and unbearable.

The treatment options will depend on the severity of the osteoarthritis. During the early stages, the standard treatment is rest, weight loss, anti inflammatory medication, physical therapy and steroid injections in some cases, and. If the arthritis becomes severe, however, a joint replacement surgery may be appropriate.

One must consider the timing of this major surgery in relation to one's age and medical conditions, recognizing that wear and loosening of implants may occur over time and revision surgery may be indicated. Thus it is important to discuss the procedure with your orthopaedic surgeon and come up with an acceptable timeline for the surgery.

Total knee replacement is a major surgery that will leave a scar on the patient's knee, which is typically about 4 to 6 inches in length but may vary based on the size of the patient's knee and leg. The surgery lasts about 2 to 3 hours and the most serious complication is infection of the joint (occurs in <1% of patients). Other complications include deep vein thrombosis (clot in the veins of the legs), which happens in up to 15% of patients, minor nerve injuries (1-2%), joint stiffness (8-23%) and prosthesis failure (2%).

Deep vein thrombosis (DVT) is often preventable, especially when the patient is actively involved in the rehabilitation process. Wearing supportive stockings and periodic elevation of the legs to promote circulation and prevent the clots from happening are good methods of minimizing the risk of DVT. In addition, the surgeon prescribes blood-thinning drugs (low molecular weight heparin), which will also help in preventing clots. Overall, this is a very safe procedure and provides the patient with great relief of symptoms and improves his/her quality of life. It may take up to eight months for complete recovery, which will require physical therapy to help reduce stiffness and improve both strength and range-of-motion.

Q | I just got injured and tore my ACL. Do I need surgery?

ACL stands for the anterior cruciate ligament. This is one of the supportive ligaments that are found inside the knee. The role of this ligament is to provide stability to the knee especially while walking uphill and doing any kind of sporting activity. The ACL is one of the most common torn ligaments, classically by twisting the leg while the knee is in a locked position (landing on the leg and quickly pivoting in the opposite direction).

The patient almost always comes into the emergency department describing a "loud pop or snap" after twisting his or her knee. The knee usually swells and becomes painful. Even though an ACL tear can be quite debilitating, it may often be accompanied by two other injuries (tear of the medical meniscus and the medial collateral ligament). If all three structures are torn, this injury is referred to as the, "Unhappy Triad."

Surgery is usually the treatment of choice for an unhappy triad injury because the patient will likely not be able to walk normally without it. On the other hand, surgery is not always needed for isolated ACL tears. If the orthopaedic surgeon feels the knee is stable and the patient is not extremely active, the patient can undergo physical therapy and will need to wear a knee brace before doing any strenuous physical activity. If the knee is unstable, however, or the patient is an athlete, surgical reconstruction will be the best treatment choice. This is usually done arthoroscopically, leaving the patient with just three one inch-long scars after the surgery. The surgeon will either use a graft from the patient's own hamstring or patellar tendon, or rarely a graft that has been properly preserved. The recovery phase is anywhere from 3-6 months and the patient will have to go to physical therapy to regain full function of the knee.

Q **My hip arthritis is so severe I can hardly walk. What are the dangers of getting a hip replacement and how can I improve my recovery?**

Hip replacement is one of the most successful and reliable orthopaedic procedures with close to 95% patient satisfaction in regaining functionality of affected hip. This is a major surgery and, again, wear and loosing of implants may also occur in hip replacement prosthesis (after several years in place). The most serious complication is infection, but dislocation of the hip prosthesis components may also occur. The operating surgeon will give specific instructions after surgery to avoid complications. The patient will most likely attend physical therapy sessions to help with the healing process which should take anywhere from 8-12 weeks.

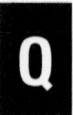

Q **What is a tennis elbow? Why did this happen to me and will I need surgery to get better?**

Tennis elbow (also known as Lateral epicondilitis) is defined as pain over the outer part of the elbow. This overuse syndrome is due to the degeneration of the Extensor Carpi Radialis Brevis (ECRB) muscle, which normally attaches to and covers a specific point on the outer part of the elbow. This muscle degeneration causes pain when flexing the wrist such as when pouring a pitcher or lifting something with the palms facing down. It's name is derived from the injury that the tennis players sustain in that area due to the repetitive nature of hitting the ball many times and causing micro tears in the tendon of this muscle at its attachement site on the elbow. There are many treatment options that are available including anti-inflammatory medications, use of a brace/ strap to reduce the tension on the elbow, steroid injections, and a possible surgery to get rid of the tissue that caused this problem in the first place. Surgery is usually withheld until the previously mentioned treatments have failed.

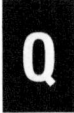

Q **My child was injured and the x-ray showed he had a "greenstick" fracture. Should he/ she have surgery or is a cast good enough to treat him?**

This is a common fracture in childhood, while the bones are still soft and young. It is called a greenstick fracture because it resembles a young green tree branch that has been bent, causing the outside of it to split without it breaking completely in half. This often happens when a child falls on outstretched hands, causing the young flexible bones of the wrist and forearm to bend and split, rather than breaking like they would if the same injury happened in an adult. No surgery is required for such cases however overcorrection maybe required (completing the fracture) along with placing a cast on the arm to immobilize the bones, thereby promoting proper healing.

Once applied, the cast is usually in place for the next 4-6weeks. The patient should be advised to raise the arm above the head on a regular basis in order to minimize the swelling that may accompany this fracture and to try to exercise the joints above and below the cast to maintain muscle strength. Children seldom require physical therapy for such injuries.

Q **I fell on my outstretched arm and broke my wrist. How can this be fixed? What if I don't want surgery?**

The majority of wrist fractures don't require surgery however one of the commonly fractured bones in the wrist is the scaphoid bone, located at the base of the thumb on the back of the hand, but it is important to note that many people refer to a fracture of a forearm as a "broken wrist." The actual location of the wrist is about an inch in from the base of the palm. The most common way to fracture a scaphoid bone is by falling on an out stretched hand. This can be very painful, or it may be a dull ache with weakness or numbness, and a bruise often develops. Whatever the sensation after such a fall, x-rays usually diagnose the fracture.

Unfortunately, not all scaphoid fractures are seen with the first set of x-rays. Surgeons often place a cast and ask the patient to come back in 7-10 days for a repeat X-ray in order to visualize the fracture. If the initial casting was successful and sufficient, evidence of bone healing will be noted and the patient will be advised to come back for regular check ups to make sure that the healing process remains on the right track. The cast usually needs to be worn for 6-12 weeks for complete healing to occur but, if no healing is noted, then surgical intervention is needed to unite the fractured scaphoid bone. This surgery involves placing a screw to hold the two fractured pieces together.

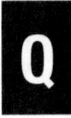

Q I have carpal tunnel syndrome and my wrists are frequently numb and tingly! Will surgery get rid of the pain and, if so, will I have to get general anesthesia?

The carpal tunnel is an anatomical pathway located at the base of the wrist, connecting the inner structures of the forearm to the hand. One nerve (the "median" nerve) and nine tendons pass through it. Compression of this nerve causes the symptoms of carpal tunnel syndrome.

In most patients the cause is unknown however it can be caused by conditions that exert pressure on the median nerve such as metabolic diseases (thyroid problems and diabetes), pregnancy, and prolonged repetitive movements like excessive use of the keyboard or sawing. Patients usually feel numbness and weakness of the hand, which may or may not be accompanied by pain, and the thumb muscles often atrophy as well. The doctor will confirm the diagnosis by performing a few very short maneuvers during the office visit.

There are several treatment options. Regular stretching and range of motion exercises for the wrist can help reduce the pain, but should be conducted with care as instructed by a physician, as to avoid further injury. If these exercises do not help, then the doctor may recommend the following options: night splints with the use of anti-inflammatory drugs, steroid injections to decrease inflammation, or carpal tunnel release surgery.

Night splint and steroid injections are the mainstay of treatment for carpal tunnel syndrome, but if the disease is severe or the patient prefers to have surgery, then surgery may be done to completely relieve the symptoms. Carpal tunnel surgery is a straightforward procedure that lasts about 30 minutes with minimal complications and leaves a 2-inch scar on the palm side of their hand. The patient usually goes home the same day.

The patient can choose between two types of anesthesia, regional or general. Most of the time, the surgeon will recommend a regional anesthesia because it is associated with decreased risks and complications. "Regional anesthesia" means that the patient's nerves are numbed so that he or she does not feel pain, but the patient remains in a semi awake state and can even observe the surgery while lying on the operating table. The main drawback to this type of anesthesia is that the patient may still have some sensation of pressure or, if the regional anesthesia is incomplete, there may be pain during the procedure. With general anesthesia, on the other hand, the patient is in deep sleep and typically does not feel or remember anything. The anesthesiologist and surgeon will discuss these options with the patient.

I'm getting really tired of my shoulder dislocating! Why does this happen? How do I prevent it? Are there any complications? Will I need surgery?

Dislocation of the shoulder occurs because the shoulder joint has the greatest range of motion in the body with relatively little structural support. The mechanism behind the dislocation involves the upper part of the arm (humerus) being dislodged from its resting place in the shoulder blade (the scapula). Shoulder dislocation requires a high-energy trauma and with older patients there may be an associated tear of the "rotator cuff," a group of structures responsible for keeping the shoulder joint stable.

Recurrent or repeat dislocations are likely to happen after the initial dislocation, because of the damage done to the shoulder joint during the initial injury. The patient's pain can sometimes be felt past the shoulder, radiating down the arm's length, and the patient is often unable to move his or her arm when the shoulder is dislocated.

Three types of dislocations are possible. An anterior (forward) dislocation is the most common type accounting for over 95% of shoulder dislocations. The most serious complication that may occur with this type is blood vessel damage, particularly the axillary artery. The second type is the posterior (backward) dislocation, usually due to severe muscle contractions as seen in electrocutions and seizures. Permanent damage to the rotator cuff muscles is a common complication of dislocation, predisposing the person to recurrent dislocations and possible fractures of the humerus itself, in which case nerves and blood vessels may be injured. The third type of dislocation is the inferior (downward) dislocation and is the least likely type, occurring in less than 1% of patients. The most common cause of this dislocation is a force from above the person's head pushing down on arm(s) fully elevated above the head, causing the shoulder to be pushed downwards and out of the joint. This dislocation has the highest complication rate because many blood vessels and nerves are located in the path of the dislocation.

When the patient presents to the ER with a dislocated shoulder, the initial mode of treatment is a "closed reduction," meaning that there is no surgery. The shoulder is just placed back into the socket through a series of movements and manipulations that are designed to place the dislocated shoulder back in its rightful place. An X-ray is taken afterwards to make sure that the shoulder is back to its anatomical location and the arm is kept in a sling for several days until an orthopaedic surgeon sees the patient for further evaluation and follow-up. If the joint is unstable and there is a strong possibility of recurrent dislocations, then surgery is required to fix the problem.

The surgery is designed to repair the damaged shoulder joint by the various means that are at the disposal of the orthopaedic surgeon. The recovery period depends on the amount of damage done to the joint and the type of procedure that the patient underwent. It may take anywhere from 4-8 months and it is very important to know what the patient can and cannot do while in the healing process. Talking to the surgeon and getting a thorough explanation of how to take care of the injured shoulder after surgery is very important and should be followed strictly. If no complications occur, the patient will usually regain close to full functionality of the shoulder and be able to return to normal activity level with few restrictions.

I have a trigger finger. What is the cause and what are my treatment options?

A trigger finger is a disorder that may affect any finger and is characterized by an often-painful catching, snapping or locking of the involved finger into a bent or flexed position. This is caused by the sheath around the tendon either tightening or thickening, and preventing the movement of the corresponding finger tendon. As a result, when the patient tries to make a fist and then straighten the fingers out, the affected finger gets stuck and needs to be manually pulled back into normal position. This manual extension of the finger is what causes the snapping sound and the pain.

Two treatment options are available. The non-surgical approach is the injection of corticosteroids into the damaged site that is effective for a few weeks to months. If the steroid injections fail, than a simple surgical procedure is done. The patient usually remains awake and the involved sheath is cut under local anesthetic to release the entrapped tendon (much like the carpal tunnel surgery). The recovery period is short and the patient should exercise the finger by fully extending it in order to get full range of motion back after the surgery.

Q

I have a ruptured Achilles' tendon. I heard that I could either get a cast or surgery. Which one should I choose?

The Achilles' tendon is the strongest and the thickest tendon in the body and it serves a vital function in our ability to walk, run, jump, and swim. Achilles' tendon rupture is one of the most common tendon ruptures and the "typical" patient is a middle-aged male between the ages of 30 and 40 who plays sports on the weekends (weekend warriors), but other groups of people also suffer from this type of tendon rupture. Most often, rupture is caused by sudden loading of the tendon while the ankle is in upward flexed position such as in missing a step or sudden jumping without the proper warm up. Other less common ways are direct injury or intense exercise after being bedridden for a long period of time. Upon presentation, the patient will usually describe hearing a loud "pop," almost like a gunshot sound, after which he or she was unable to walk.

Although Achilles' tendon ruptures are usually fairly easy to diagnose clinically, the surgeon may decide to take some x-rays, ultrasound, or MRI's to precisely see if it is a complete tear or just a partial tear. There are two treatment options available: the surgical and the non-surgical. Usually, the non-surgical approach is selected for minor tears, less active patients, or those who have other medical problems that would prevent them from undergoing surgery. This approach involves placing a hard cast or specialized boots on the foot and the ankle in such a way as to bring the two ruptured ends together so that the healing can take place (much like the casting of broken bones).

For more active patients, many surgeons recommend surgery, which can be either an open procedure (larger scar) or less often a percutaneous one (smaller scar). Surgery is believed to result in a stronger repair with less re-rupture than a cast or boot, but some recent studies have shown that there is no difference between the surgical and the non-surgical approaches. Hence, although surgery carries greater risk of complication, the major difference between these two procedures is the recovery time, with the surgical approach having a shorter recovery time and possibly a lower re-rupture rate.

When rehabilitating the ruptured tendon, the first phase begins with range of motion stretching to allow the ankle to get used to movement again. The second phase involves the application of gradual weight on the affected ankle in order to start building strength in the tendon to get it ready for physical activity. Discuss the treatment options with your orthopaedic surgeon for best results.

NEUROSURGERY

// See Disclaimer on page 1 of this book before reading this chapter.

Authors:

RADOMIR KOSANOVIC, MS-III
St. George's University School of Medicine

Editors:

PARHAM YASHAR, M.D.
Endovascular Fellow, Department of Neurological Surgery
University at Buffalo – SUNY
Millard Fillmore Gates Hospital, Buffalo, NY

JONATHAN MAREHBIAN, MS-IV
St. George's University School of Medicine

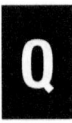

Q **I have a herniated disc: Is surgery necessary? How effective is herniated disc surgery? Will I regain my function back without pain?**

Disc herniation is a common reason for back pain. Surgery is not immediately recommended for everyone, however, until a number of conservative, less aggressive treatments are tried first. Some examples include rest, over-the-counter drugs (i.e. anti-inflammatory medications, steroids, muscle relaxants, and pain medications), spinal manipulations, and epidural or spinal injections. Depending on the patient's symptoms, if these do not work then surgery is often recommended.

Discectomy would typically be the surgery done in this situation. Discectomy is the removal of material from a herniated disc, which was compressing either the spinal cord or a spinal nerve nearby. Such compression can lead to various neurological symptoms, like weakness, tingling, and pain in various parts of the body (usually the legs). The relief of symptoms (the most common symptom is pain) is not straightforward. The recovery depends on the amount and extent of damage caused by the herniated disc. In some patients, simple removal of the debris around the spinal nerve will relieve the problem. In other patients in whom the spinal injury is greater, the recovery can take weeks to months. Unfortunately, some patients never find full relief of pain or other symptoms after the surgery.

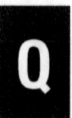

Q Can surgery improve my Parkinson's disease?

Parkinson's disease (PD) affects 4.5 million Americans. It is a progressive degenerative neurological disease that affects the central nervous system (the brain and spinal cord). PD results from a degeneration of a specific type of cell in the substantia nigra of the brain that produces dopamine. PD impairs motor skills (movement), memory, speech and other functions. It leads to rigidity (called "cog-wheel" rigidity) of the arms and legs, resting tremors (fine tremors seen in the hands), slowing of movements and shuffling of the feet while walking (also known as festinating gait).

The most common treatment is medical, with the use of medications that mimic the actions of the neurotransmitter dopamine, whose actions are therefore impaired with this disease. If medical management is not effective, however, there are a few different surgical options: Deep Brain Stimulation (DBS), Pallidotomy and Thalamotomy.

DBS works by implanting wire electrodes in the brain to stimulate electrical signals necessary for normal brain signaling and control of movements in the PD patient. This treatment is often effective at controlling the disabling tremor and improving both balance and walking ability, and is most helpful in those patients who have shown improvement with medical management. Pallidotomy (another surgical technique) is destruction of the globus pallidus, which is a small region within the brain that is important in controlling movement. Thalamotomy, a third type of surgery, is destruction of another a specific small area in the brain called the thalamus (also involved in the control of movement). Both Pallidotomy and Thalamotomy are older methods of a more destructive nature. Today, the preferred method for treating PD is with DBS and medications.

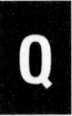

Q

I recently suffered from a mini stroke or TIA (transient ischemic attack); will surgery help to prevent a full-blown stroke from taking place?

Typically the treatment for prevention of strokes is medical, with strict control of blood pressure, cholesterol, blood sugar, salt intake, and the minimization of lifestyle-oriented risk factors like smoking, alcohol intake, and obesity. In people with heart disease or arrhythmias, other medications may be necessary. A TIA (often called "mini-stroke") is a temporary loss of neurologic function that returns within 24 hours and shows no signs of permanent brain damage. A stroke results in permanent brain damage resulting from death of brain tissue.

Stroke can be classified as either a hemorrhagic stroke (a burst blood vessel bleeding in the brain) or an ischemic stroke (clogged blood vessel resulting in lack of blood flow and oxygen to a portion of the brain).

There is a third type of bleeding into the brain that results from a ruptured aneurysm, called subarachnoid hemorrhage, which can often be confused with a stroke. Unlike strokes, which present with symptoms of one-sided weakness, confusion, facial drooping, and/ or an inability to speak properly, subarachnoid hemorrhages typically present with patients complaining of "the worst headache in their life," classically occurring and worsening rapidly.

Ischemic strokes occur when there's decreased blood flow to a particular region of the brain. This can be due to a variety of causes: (1) slow cholesterol buildup resulting in a blockade of one the main arteries in the neck (carotid artery), (2) due to these cholesterol plaques breaking off and suddenly lodging themselves in and blocking off an artery within the brain or (3) when a clot that forms in the heart in patients with irregular heart rhythm lodges itself in the brain. In any case, it is critically important to seek medical help immediately. The sooner treatment is started the better the outcome will be. Many people recover some level of function after a stroke, especially, if the symptoms are recognized early and they are treated early.

Surgery is usually not used to treat an acute stroke, although it maybe indicated for a hemorrhagic stroke or a recent blockade of a carotid artery. Researchers are learning that TIA's are the most reliable warning signs of a future full-blown stroke. Between 10-50% of strokes are preceded by a TIA and, if not treated, about 1/3 of all patients that suffer from a TIA will experience a stroke within 5 years. The goal in surgery is to reestablish adequate blood supply to injured brain tissue or to relieve pressure caused by an actively bleeding blood vessel. Other, more modern, treatment options for acute strokes are those within the field of endovascular treatments. These include attempts at opening up the blockages by using a combination of small wires, catheters, stents, and injections of various medications within the vessels themselves in order to re-establish blood flow to vital parts of the brain.

There are multiple factors that must be taken into account before surgery can be considered: the patient's age, the patient's known or understood wishes, prior state of health, known medical conditions, as well as the exact type and location of the mini stroke or TIA he or she had. Hence, it is extremely important to provide the hospital physicians with a thorough medical history so that the safest and most effective treatment can be administered.

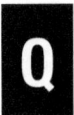

Q **My spouse has hydrocephalus. Will surgery be able to reverse it?**

Hydrocephalus is the accumulation of too much fluid (called, "cerebral spinal fluid," or CSF) within the fluid-filled spaces of the brain or skull ("ventricles"), squeezing the brain against the hard skull. The condition is caused by either too much CSF production (rare) or, more commonly, by a blockage in the normal outflow or drainage of this fluid from the skull, resulting in high pressures inside the skull. CSF is a clear fluid that functions in the buoyancy, protection, chemical stability and prevention of blood loss from the brain tissue. Most of the reported cases occur later in life, although this condition can occur in infants and children too. The most common complaint is headache. The headaches may not be long lasting and are relieved with changing the position of the head. Other symptoms may include a nausea, vomiting, loss of balance, blurred vision, loss of bladder and/or bowel control, or other neurological deficits. Depending on the cause, if left untreated, it can progress to lethargy, coma, or even death.

Hydrocephalus can lead to many neurological problems, including sudden death, and surgery is the best treatment. There are two types of surgical procedures that can help treat hydrocephalus. The most common type is a small tube, called a "shunt" or "bypass," inserted inside the brain to drain excess CSF out of the skull in order to relieve the excess pressure from the increased amount of CSF. The shunt drains the excess CSF into the abdomen (or other locations). There may be an option to remove whatever is obstructing the drainage of fluid, but this option is not always possible. In specific cases, a small camera can be used to bypass the blockage of CSF in the brain, from one compartment to another, to allow its reabsorption ("endoscopic third ventriculostomy"). It is important to note that correcting hydrocephalus sooner rather than later will decrease the chances of brain damage developing.

Q Will I lose my hearing after Schwannoma surgery?

A schwannoma is a tumor of the cells of the protective sheath that covers nerves of the peripheral nervous system (nerves outside the brain and spinal cord). The most common location for a Schwannoma is within the skull but outside the brain, itself. This tumor is attached to the nerves that are responsible for our sense of hearing. The most common early symptom of a schwannomas is tinnitus, or "ringing in the ears." Other frequent symptoms include hearing loss, imbalance, or dizziness.

Two main factors important in the treatment of this type of non-cancerous tumor are its size and precise location. These factors will determine the type of treatment that will be offered in order to treat the tumor—whether it is surgery or another treatment. Also part of the work-up of a schwannomas is a hearing test called an audiogram. Simply put, if the patient has the ability to hear before surgery, the surgeon will aim to preserve this hearing after surgery. However, if the patient's hearing has been significantly compromised, it will frequently be destroyed (intentionally) at the benefit of removing the entire tumor during the surgery. Typically, patients that present with larger tumors already have some form of hearing loss. Regardless, surgery is still the recommended treatment for large tumors because the tumor, if not removed, will continue to compress other structures within the skull.

Q I suffer from Trigeminal neuralgia. Will surgery stop the pain?

Trigeminal neuralgia (TN), also known as "tic douloureux," is severe, sudden, painful electric-like shocks that affect the face. The most frequent cause is believed to be due to compression of the Trigeminal nerve, which supplies sensation to the face, by engorgement of surrounding blood vessels. Pain is felt when patients chew food, laugh, talk, or even touch their faces. In some patients multiple sclerosis (MS), these symptoms can be present on both sides of the face. Initially, TN is treated with medications like carbamazepine (Trade name: tegretol), but if this does not work a common surgical procedure, Microvascular Decompression (MVD) surgery may be recommended.

The New England Journal of Medicine published a report in 1996, which showed that the initial success rate for complete relief of pain was 82% with MVD; partial relief was seen in 16%. After a 10-year follow up (2006), 68% had excellent or good relief and 32% had recurrent symptoms.

Other treatment options include radiosurgery (focused radiation to the nerve), injection of glycerol or alcohol (called "percutaneous trimeminal rhizotomy), or with a balloon compression of the trigeminal nerve bundle (ganglion).

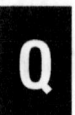

Q **I am told I suffer from spinal stenosis. Can the stenosis be fixed with surgery?**

Spinal stenosis (SS) occurs when the canal around the spinal cord narrows and compresses the spinal cord and/or spinal nerves. SS is relatively common in older populations. The vertebral bones that make up the spinal column surrounding the spinal cord begin to degenerate, leading to a thickening of the surrounding structures (joints, bone, ligaments) resulting in the compression of the spinal cord itself.

Spinal stenosis can occur at any part of the spinal column but the most common are the cervical (neck) and lumbar (lower back) portions. The symptoms vary depending on the location of the stenosis but patients usually present with numbness, weakness, neck or shoulder pain (only if the cervical segment is involved), pain in the legs or back (typical of lumbar spinal stenosis) and loss of bowel and bladder control when severe.

Laminectomy, a surgical procedure in which parts of one or more vertebral bones are removed to relieve pressure on the spinal cord or spinal nerve(s), is the treatment of choice in most cases. There is still some controversy between the benefits of both surgical and non-surgical procedures, however, because studies show positive effects of each treatment. It is best to talk to your neurosurgeon to get the best treatment for you.

PLASTIC, RECONSTRUCTIVE, & HAND SURGERY

// See Disclaimer on page 1 of this book before reading this chapter.

Authors:

JULIE FERRAUIOLA, MS-IV
St. George's University School of Medicine

Editors:

NADEEM A. CHAUDHRY, M.D., F.A.C.S.
Chief, Division of Plastic Surgery
The Brooklyn Hospital Center, Brooklyn, NY

Q Why is it called "plastic surgery"?

Yes, some plastic surgeries do use silicone and other prosthetic implant materials, but that is not the reason it is called plastic surgery. The word "plastic" comes from the Greek word, "plastikos," which means, "to mold or shape." The aim of many plastic surgeries is to mold and reshape the body into the desired form. Plastic surgery has deep historical roots with the first mention of the treatment of nasal injuries appearing in the Edwin Smith Surgical Papyrus dated circa 3000 BCE and a description of a method of transferring skin from the forehead and cheek to reconstruct a nose appearing in 400 BCE in an Indian encyclopedia (Samhita) by Sushruta, who is widely believed to be the first plastic surgeon.

Q How do I find a plastic surgeon?

Choosing a plastic surgeon may seem like a daunting task, but it is not a decision to be taken lightly. Opening up the yellow pages to "plastic surgeons" does not guarantee that the surgeon listed is indeed a board certified plastic surgeon.

The following agencies are a good place to start looking:

- American Board of Plastic Surgery (ABPS)
- American Society of Plastic Surgeons (ASPS)
- American Society for Aesthetic Plastic Surgery (ASAPS)
- American Board of Facial Plastic & Reconstructive Surgery (ABFPRS)
- American Association of Facial Plastic & Reconstructive Surgery (AAFPRS)
- Canadian Society of Plastic Surgeons

All of these organizations have extensive consumer resources and information as well as a database of members. Membership to these organizations ensures that the plastic surgeon is board certified and has had extensive training and experience with plastic surgery procedures.

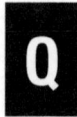 **I already have a surgeon in mind. What are a few things I can do to find out if he or she is a good match for me?**

• **Check the surgeon's board certification**, either directly from the surgeon or from the organizations listed above.

• **Ask where your surgery will take place.** Most procedures can be safely performed in an office-based facility, but not all offices are "accredited facilities" for surgical procedures. By choosing a surgeon who operates in an accredited facility you can be sure the facility has regular inspections and reports to State regulatory agencies.

• **Inquire about follow-up care.** Be sure to find out what kind of follow-up visits you can expect and the doctor's policy on revision surgery should it be necessary.

• **Check the surgeon's website,** if he or she has one.

• Ask the surgeon for "informed consent."

• **For cosmetic procedures,** check the surgeon's profile; most will have albums of their past work in their offices.

• **Recognize that the possibility** exists that complications will arise and/or that additional surgery to further improve your results may be an option for you.

Q My doctor says he can do the procedure in his office's surgical suite, is it safe?

The growth of office-based surgery has seen dramatic increases since 1990 when it accounted for 1.2 million procedures per year. It is now estimated that outpatient surgery accounts for up to 25% of operative procedures performed each year. To ensure that the surgical facility meets acceptable safety standards make sure it is accredited by a national or state recognized accrediting agency such as the American Association for Ambulatory Surgery Facilities (AAAASF), Accreditation Association for Ambulatory Health Care (AAAHC), or the Joint Commission on the Accreditation of Healthcare Organizations (JCAHO).

There is a long track record of safety for plastic surgery procedures performed by board certified plastic surgeons in accredited facilities; a 1997 survey based on more than 400,000 procedures found that serious complications occurred in less than one-half percent of cases and the mortality rate was extremely low, one in 57,000. It was found that the risk rate for serious complications in an accredited office-based facility is comparable to a hospital ambulatory surgical center or a freestanding surgical center. To find out the accreditation status of a facility contact AAAASF at www.aaaasf.org, AAAHC at www.aahc.org or JCAHO at www.jcaho.org.

Keep in mind that procedures done in foreign countries could be dangerous and seeking help for complications upon your return could be difficult.

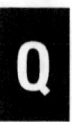

Q **What should I know about the different kinds of anesthesia used in plastic surgery?**

There are many different kinds of anesthesia and an informed patient should know a little about each kind and ask which one will be used during the procedure. The two most common types used in plastic surgery procedures are general anesthesia and monitored anesthetic care (MAC).

General anesthesia is defined as, "a controlled state of unconsciousness accompanied by loss of protective airway reflexes." General anesthesia has three distinct phases: induction, maintenance, and emergence. The induction phase is when the patient loses consciousness and is usually achieved with intravenous medications.

General anesthesia requires control of the patient's airway and often, mechanical ventilation. This can be achieved by either passing a tube into the airway beyond the vocal cords (intubation) or with a laryngeal mask airway (LMA) that is placed above the vocal cords. The most common complaint post-operatively in regards to airway protection is a sore throat.

After the induction phase the anesthesiologist begins the maintenance phase. During this time the patient's oxygen saturation, blood pressure, heart rate and rhythm, respiratory rate, and temperature are closely monitored and a combination of drugs is administered to maintain the unconscious state. This can be achieved through either inhaled or intravenous anesthetics.

Inhaled anesthetics, while low in cost, can cause significant post-operative nausea and vomiting when compared to intravenous anesthesia, like continuous infusion propofol. However, the times to extubation and return of cognitive function are longer with intravenous anesthesia. Emergence, or "waking up" is when the concentration of the anesthetics is lowered to allow the patient to regain a conscious state. During this time the patient's vital signs remain closely monitored and, once the patient regains the reflexes necessary to protect his or her own airway the endotracheal tube or LMA is removed. The patient continues to be monitored carefully in the post-operative period for any signs of hypertension, low oxygen, pain, nausea and vomiting.

Monitored anesthetic care is a technique that uses a combination of local anesthetic (an injection of numbing medication at the surgical site) and intravenous analgesic and sedative drugs to produce a "conscious sedation" whereby the patient has a minimally depressed level of consciousness, but continues to breath on his or her own.

The type of anesthesia used largely depends on the procedure and the judgment of the anesthesiologist and surgeon. Long or complicated procedures typically call for general anesthesia, while shorter procedures may be done with conscious sedation. Both types of anesthesia are safe in the ambulatory office setting and a recent study showed no significant differences between the two in terms of recovery time, sensitivity to pain or safety.

Q   Will my surgery results last forever, or will I need more surgery?

Certain procedures are more likely to need additional procedures down the road. As we age, our bodies change and skin becomes less elastic and gravity always wins. Breast implants will often need to be replaced or revised. Breast implants can deflate, become infected or encapsulated, or go south the way natural breasts do, requiring additional surgery. Liposuction results can be reversed with weight gain and the fat may distribute in unsightly ways. Facelifts require life-long sun protection to maintain a youthful appearance and may require additional surgeries to "refresh" the results.

One must always recognize the possibility of complications arising during and/or after surgery, but the risks of each complication are unique to both you and the procedure you are having done, so you should discuss them with your physician. When contemplating a procedure, have clear realistic expectations for the results and discuss them with your plastic surgeon. Also make sure to discuss how long you can expect your results to last.

Q **What is the recovery like? And, how is it different from recovery for other types of surgery?**

Plastic surgery consists of many different procedures on various parts of the body, so it follows that recovery varies depending on the procedure and the patient. Surgeries that involve large areas of the body or require extensive movement of tissue and muscle, such as liposuction or breast augmentation, generally tend to have greater discomfort in the post-operative period and will take longer before you can resume your normal daily activities.

Regardless of the procedure, you can expect to have bandages over the area that was operated on and you will need to return to the office in a few days to have them changed or removed. The first few days you can expect pain and swelling, this is your body's healing response kicking in. Some procedures will require the use of a drain, where one end of a small tube is left inside the body and it is attached to a little plastic bulb that is outside the body and collects the fluid that builds up. The fluid will often look like light colored blood, and the amount of fluid drained will usually decrease as time goes on.

Most patients will require assistance for the first two days after surgery, longer if they have small children to care for. Each procedure will have its own healing time, which should be outlined by the plastic surgeon. Regular exercise and vigorous activities are usually prohibited during the first two weeks post-operatively to decrease the risks of bleeding, swelling and bruising.

Q | What's the difference between plastic and reconstructive surgery?

The goal of plastic surgery, also called cosmetic surgery, is to change the patient's appearance by altering parts of the body that function normally to improve self-esteem and body satisfaction. Most cosmetic surgeries are considered elective.

Reconstructive surgery differs in that the part of the body being operated on is abnormal in structure or function due to congenital defects, injury, tumors, or disease. The main goal is the restoration of form and function.

There is some overlap between the two, where a cosmetic procedure is can also be a reconstructive one depending on the patient's situation. For example, if a breast reduction or lift is performed because a woman wants smaller, perkier breasts it is a cosmetic procedure, if it is performed to relieve severe back pain then it is a reconstructive procedure.

UROLOGY

// See Disclaimer on page 1 of this book before reading this chapter.

Authors:

RADOMIR KOSANOVIC, MS-III
St. George's University School of Medicine

Editors:

Y. SAMUEL LITVIN M.D.
Assistant Clinical Professor, Urology
Drexel University School of Medicine, Philadelphia, PA

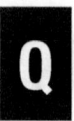

Q

Will I still be able to have sex, even If I undergo surgery for penile cancer?

Penile cancer is a malignant tumor that develops from the skin cells of the penis. It is a rare type of cancer that affects mainly elderly men between the ages of 60 and 80 and occurs almost exclusively in uncircumcised males. In 2008, the American Cancer Society estimated there were 1250 new patients in the United States per year.

Penile cancer generally presents with an ulcerated lesion (sore) that becomes an infiltrating (deeper) ulcer, which can then become either a papillary (small nipple-like projection) or verrucous (wart like) lesion. The most common sites for cancer to develop on the penis are the glans penis (head of the penis) and the prepuce (foreskin). The treatment is surgery.

The amount of tissue that must be surgically removed can determine both the degree of remaining sexual function and the ability to aim the urinary stream. Multiple studies have evaluated sexual function and satisfaction after surgery to remove this type of cancer. These studies have found mixed results, ranging from about 30% loss of sexual function to higher than 70%. In addition to the physical bodily changes following this type a surgery, some researchers believe that psychological factors play a significant role in loss of function.

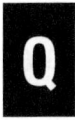

Q **I was just diagnosed with testicular cancer. If I have surgery to remove that testicle will I still be able to have children?**

The occurrence of testicular cancer has increased in the last 40 years, more so in northern European populations. Although the reason for this increase is unknown, testicular cancers are known to account for about 1% of all cancers in men and can affect both testicles. Testicular germ cell tumors (GCT) make up 90-95% of the malignant testicular tumors. The tumor occurs most frequently in men between the ages of 20 and 40.

Patients with GCT are at increased risk of developing decreased testosterone production. Leydig cells, which are located inside of the testes, are responsible for the production of testosterone. Testosterone is needed for the normal production of sperm. Hence, a person who has a testicle removed will have decreased sperm production. If one testicle is not removed, there may be some leftover testosterone production but the amount of testosterone the man produces and the functionality of his sperm must be evaluated on an individual basis.

When testicular cancer is diagnosed early, outcomes are better. In 2009, the American Cancer Society estimated there were 8400 new cases of testicular cancer, of which 380 led to death. Hence, early detection may save a man's life and allow for the man to donate his sperm to be "frozen" so that they may be used for artificial insemination at a later date.

Patients sometimes have pre-existing infertility, and those with an atrophic testicle on the opposite side should be biopsied at the time of surgery. Patients who are fertile at the time of diagnosis are generally recommended to bank sperm in case they do not regain fertility after treatment. Modern chemotherapy, if needed, allows the return of fertility in a significant percentage of previously fertile men. If Retroperitoneal Lymph Node Dissection (RPLND) is required, a sizable percentage of previously fertile men will have an inability to ejaculate due to nerve damage.

Q **I was just diagnosed with an enlarged prostate (AKA Benign Prostatic Hyperplasia or "BPH"). Will surgery allow me to pee normally again?**

BPH is caused by an increase in size of the prostate. It usually affects men starting after the age of 50, more commonly in white men than in other races. The prostate increases in size by a process called hyperplasia (increase in the number of the cells) of the prostate. Unfortunately, the urethra – the tube that allows for urine to flow from the bladed out of the penis – is surrounded and then compressed by this enlarged prostate.

Compression of the urethra leads to lower urinary tract symptoms: urgency, frequency, nocturia, hesitancy in voiding, poor flow, dribbling, and incomplete voiding. If left untreated, BPH can then lead to other complications, like urinary flow problems, kidney problems, and urinary tract infections (UTIs).

Surgery is not the first choice for treatment and medications are often prescribed instead. If medical therapy does not work, then surgery becomes the treatment of choice and the urinary symptoms improve for most people, but some complications are possible. The current "gold standard" procedure is called Transurethral Resection of the Prostate (TURP) and it has a very high rate of success with low complication rates. A small percentage of previously potent patients have erectile dysfunction afterward (<5%) and an even smaller percentage (<1%) have urinary continence problems.

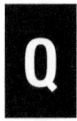 **I have really painful kidney stones. Do I need surgery and, if I opt for it, will surgery prevent the stones from reappearing?**

Kidney stones are made up of different components, or materials. The most common type of stone is made from calcium oxalate or calcium phosphate. Less common stones are composed of uric acid, magnesium ammonium phosphate, or cysteine. Each type of stone formation is due to a different cause.

Surgery used to be the mainstay for treatment of kidney stones, but has been replaced by less invasive treatments. The best treatment options are generally determined by the size and location of the stone within the urinary tract, the presence of associated infection, and whether pain can be managed with medication while an attempt at stone passage takes place. Common treatments are shock wave lithotripsy, ureteroscopy or percutaneous nephrolithotomy, all designed to identify, break-up, and flush out the stones so that they are no longer obstructing the urinary tract. Unfortunately, kidney stones recur in 30-50% of patients within 5 years.

For patients with kidney stones, long-term prevention focuses on dietary changes and a higher fluid intake. If these tactics do not work, then medications are prescribed to lower urine calcium (thiazide diuretics), block uric acid production (allopurinol), or to control other aspects of stone formation.

Q I was told that because I have varicocele, I might be infertile. Can surgery prevent this?

Varicocele is an abnormal enlargement of the testicular veins (called, "pampiniform venous plexus"). It occurs in about 15-20% of the male population at some point in their life and is found in 19-41% of the men seeking help for infertility. The exact reason that links varicocele and infertility together is still not fully understood, but there are a few hypotheses as to why there appears to be a relationship between the two.

The main hypothesis suggests that there is an increase in temperature of the testicle because of poor circulation, which causes problems with sperm formation. Using a new technique called, "sperm chromatin dispersion test (SCD)," sperm DNA was analyzed for fragmentation and it was found that there is a higher frequency of sperm cells with fragmented (pieces) of DNA in the ejaculate of varicocele patients when compared to non-varicocele patients. This increase in fragmented DNA is believed to contribute to infertility.

Surgery can be performed to repair the varicocele and increase the chances of fertility. The procedure is called microsurgical subinguinal varicocele repair (MSVR). Studies have confirmed that the MSVR technique is effective, showing that after the procedure, a significant percentage of patients are able to produce functional sperm.

Q Will circumcision decrease my chances for getting HIV?

Circumcision is the removal of the foreskin (prepuce) of the penis. The foreskin has multiple functions. It maintains a moist environment for the head of the penis and houses immune system cells (Langerhans cells) that are ready to fight any potential sexually transmitted infections.

Unfortunately, the human immunodeficiency virus (HIV) infects immune system cells like the Langerhans cells. The foreskin is also the first part of the penis that comes into contact with the partner during intercourse. Removal of the foreskin means there will be less chance of HIV infection because there will be fewer immune system cells immediately exposed to the virus during sexual activity, but it does not lead to immunity and safe sex practices should still be adhered to.

Recent studies have shown that circumcision decreases the transmission of HIV, leading to as much as a 60-70% protective effect against heterosexual transmission of HIV. Long-term studies (evaluating patients over two decades) showed that circumcision lead to a 55% decrease in the risk of acquiring HIV infections. In addition to its protective effects against HIV, circumcision has been shown to reduce the rate of Herpes and Human Papillomavirus (HPV) transmission. The World Health Organization now endorses male circumcision as an effective way to prevent the spread of HIV.

HIV, Herpes, and HPV infections are still diseases that affect all ages, races, religions and sexual preferences.

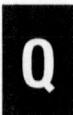

Q **I do not like to wear condoms, but I don't want my wife / girlfriend to get pregnant. Can a vasectomy cause any complications? Is it reversible?**

A vasectomy is a process where the vas deferens (a slender tube that carries sperm from the testicles to the urethra) is cut or tied. It is considered a safe and reliable means to prevent pregnancy. Worldwide over 42 million couples have used this method as a form of birth control. Studies have shown transient re-appearance of sperm after vasectomy in 0.8-2.4% of patients. A vasectomy should NEVER be done on anyone who isn't sure he (and his partner) wants PERMANENT sterilization. While a partner's agreement to this is not legally required, it is advisable.

The complications of a vasectomy are very rare, but include the following:

1. Failure of the operation to make the man sterile, which can lead to an unwanted pregnancy.
2. Postoperative hematoma (bruising) with or without infection.
3. Chronic pain in the scrotum
4. Atrophy (decrease in the size) of the testicle.

Although a vasectomy is technically reversible, it can be a difficult microsurgical procedure, and is expensive and is not covered by insurance. Success rates (measured in terms of pregnancy) decline with time, but generally do not exceed 70%. This further suggests that the procedure be considered PERMANENT sterilization, and all patients are so advised.

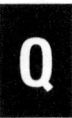 **I smoke cigarettes. Is it true that smoking can lead to urinary bladder cancer? How can this cancer be treated?**

In the United States bladder cancer is the 4th most common cancer in men and the 9th most common cancer in women. The most important risk factor is believed to be cigarette smoke, accounting for about 50% of cases. It has been found that cigarettes contain a chemical called 4-aminobiphenyl (4-ABP), a human-bladder carcinogen (cancer causing agent). 4-ABP causes DNA damage, which leads to mutations in the urinary bladder cells and, ultimately, bladder cancer (specifically called transitional cell carcinoma or TCC).

Smoking not only affects the smoker but also everyone close by that is breathing the same air (2nd hand smoke). Smokers have a two-fold greater chance of getting TCC than non-smokers. Other things can also cause bladder cancer, including: industrial chemicals (aromatic dyes, paints, solvents, leather dust, inks, combustion products, rubber and textiles), the bacterium Schistosoma hematobium, genetic disorders, drugs like cyclophosphamide, and chronic urinary tract infections.

The specific type of treatment often depends on the stage of the cancer and the extent to which it has spread. Treatments for bladder cancer include both medical (chemotherapy) and surgical treatments. Most bladder cancers are low grade and superficial (limited to the lining or "mucosa" of the bladder) and can be managed without the need to remove the bladder. However, if needed, the surgery of choice for TCC is called radical cystectomy (RC) with bilateral pelvic lymph node excision. Unfortunately, all types have a tendency to recur because all of the bladder cells have been exposed to whatever carcinogens have contributed to its formation, so speak with your urologist to decide on the best treatment for you.

Q **I recently got penile warts. What treatment options are there for me and are there consequences of never getting treated at all?**

Genital warts are most commonly due to the human papillomavirus (HPV). In the United States, the annual prevalence of HPV is estimated at 1% of the sexually active people, with more than 500,000 new cases being reported each year. The highest reported numbers are found between the ages of 20-29 years old.

There are over 100 different strains of HPV of which 40 are related to anogenital tract infections, like those found on a penis. Specifically, types 6 and 11, account for about 90% of all anogenital warts. Genital warts are typically not life threatening (although some can cause penile cancer) but they can have psychological effects. Hence, there is usually no immediate danger to men and women (note that the high risk types HPV 16 and 18 have been shown to lead to cervical cancer), but since it is sexually transmitted, the result of not getting treated is the potential for transmission of the virus to all future sexual partners.

HPV can be removed by many techniques, all of which are equally effective: surgical excision, loop electrosurgical excision, laser treatment and treatment with drugs (trichloroacetic acid, imiquimod and podophyllin). Warts often recur within the first 6 months of treatment, so multiple sessions are often needed. As with most sexually transmitted infections, abstinence is considered the most effective way to prevent infection. Also vaccination is available against types 6, 11, 16, and 18; it is recommended for all women ages 9 to 26.

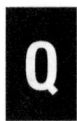

Q | I suffer from Peyronies disease (bent penis disease). Will surgery lead to a return of normal function for my penis?

Peyronies disease (PD) is a connective tissue disorder that leads to increased growth of the tough fibrous tissue inside the soft tissue of the penis. Within the penis there is a fibrous layer called the tunica albuginea, which surrounds the corpora cavernosa (the soft spongy-like erectile tissue which makes up majority of the shaft of the penis). During arousal, the corpora cavernosa normally becomes engorged with blood and leads to an erect penis – a process often disrupted in patients with PD.

In PD, the deformed tough tunical albuginea does not allow the penis to take on its normal erect shape, leading to a bend or curve in the shaft. PD is an acquired condition that is believed to be due to minor penile trauma and subsequent improper healing (increased fibrosis within the penile tissue). Penile curving during an erection can lead to pain and erectile dysfunction (ED). ED is estimated to be present in 30% of all cases of PD.

Surgery is available for patients after they have tried medical therapy without success, but most patients with Peyronie's Disease do not have deformities severe enough to require surgery. In order to need surgery, patients should have a curvature severe enough to impair normal intercourse, or cause pain during intercourse. Surgical treatment, if needed, is tailored on a case-by-case basis due to individual variation in the location and extent of plaque and deformity. There are many different surgical approaches for PD: plication, graft-based, and prosthetic techniques. The goal of surgery is to make the two sides of the penis equal, either by lengthening or shortening one side. If lengthening is desired, then a graft must be used. Each case is individualized, so you should talk to your urologist to see which method is best for you.

OPHTHALMOLOGY: EYE SURGERY

// See Disclaimer on page 1 of this book before reading this chapter.

Authors:

JAMIE SCHAEFER, MS-III
St. George's University School of Medicine

Editors:

DOUGLAS R. LAZZARO MD, FAAO, FACS
Professor and Chairman, Ophthalmology
SUNY Downstate Medical Center, Brooklyn, NY
The Richard C. Troutman MD Distinguished Chair in Ophthalmology and Ophthalmic Microsurgery

Q I am very nervous about my eye surgery, will I be awake during my operation?

Most eye surgeries are performed while the patient is awake. Local anesthesia is the most common anesthetic method. The physician may use topical numbing eye drops and/or retrobulbar (behind the globe of the eye) and peribulbar (in an area surrounding the eye) anesthetic techniques in order to eliminate the sensation of pain as well as to immobilize the extraocular muscles, the muscles around the eye that allow for movement of the eye. Patients frequently receive intraocular (directly into the eye) medication for cataract surgery.

With the administration of mild sedatives, most patients doze off during the actual procedure and remember very little about the actual surgery.

General anesthesia may be used in some cases; surgeries on children, excessive orbital and eye trauma, orbital tumors, corneal transplants, and for apprehensive patients.

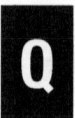

Q Can I wear eye makeup around the time of my eye surgery?

After the usage of makeup there is a high probability of that makeup to retain some bacteria, such as benign bacteria that everyone has on their skin, which under normal conditions would not affect the person who uses it. However, with surgery, you may have breaks in the skin, incisions in the eye, or any other intended trauma to or around the eye that the matter of the makeup may irritate directly or that the presence of bacteria may infect.

To reduce the risk of irritation and infection it is suggested to keep the area around the eye clean before the surgery in addition to refraining from wearing makeup for approximately a week post-surgery to allow the area of the eye worked on during surgery to heal properly.

Q Can I drive myself to get my eye surgery done?

Even though the most common eye surgeries are outpatient procedures it is highly suggested to have another person drive you home. The procedure you endure may have a direct effect on your vision, which is an unsafe condition to drive in. You may receive a patch on the operated eye making it difficult to see properly, as well as the possible effect and duration the anesthesia may have on you.

Q **What happens if I blink during my eye surgery?**

You don't have to worry about blinking or any other accidental movements during your surgery. The surgeon either tapes the eyelid back or uses a device (lid speculum) which is precisely placed to hold back the lid. This may cause a little discomfort but usually does not hurt.

Q   What types of laser eye surgeries are there?

Laser eye surgery is considered as a means of correction for people with vision problems caused by refractive errors such as hyperopia (farsightedness), myopia (nearsightedness), or astigmatism. The more common of the laser procedures include LASIK and PRK eye surgery. With LASIK eye surgery, or laser assisted in situ keratomileusis, a thin flap in the eye's cornea is created, then folded back so that the surgeon can use a laser to remove some of the corneal tissues underneath. After the desired tissue is removed, the flap is laid back in place.

For those with mild to moderate refractive vision problems or thin corneas, PRK surgery may be used. This procedure utilizes a laser to remove tissue from the cornea's surface.

Q What exactly is LASIK and am I a candidate for it?

LASIK (laser-assisted in situ keratomileusis) is a surgical procedure performed by an ophthalmologist using a beam of light, the laser, to reshape the cornea. The cornea is transparent tissue that covers the front part of the eye; its purpose is to transmit and help focus light entering the eye so that one may see.

The surgery begins when the doctor creates a thin circular flap in the cornea, which is then folded back so that the other corneal tissue beneath may be focused on for the remainder of the surgery.

The laser beam is directed to remove trace amounts of corneal tissue to correct visual irregularities such as to flatten the cornea for those with nearsightedness, to steepen the cornea for those with farsightedness who have too flat a cornea, or to smooth irregularities in the cornea into a more normal shape to correct astigmatism.

After the correction is made, the thin circular flap is then placed back over the area where the corneal tissue was removed.

Q **If I decide to get laser eye surgery, what are the worst complications that could happen to me?**

Although serious vision-reducing complications are uncommon in laser eye surgery, any procedure involving the eye has the risk of loss of vision to that eye or may even cause impairment to your vision that may not be corrected by glasses, contact lenses, or surgery. Such complications include the development of double vision, glare, or halos around light. Even if your visual sharpness improves, there is a risk of not seeing as well at night or in low contrast situations.

Some people who undergo laser eye surgery develop severe dry eye syndrome as a result of not being able to produce enough tears. This condition may be temporary or permanent, but the effects may be lessened with the use of lubricating eye drops or by the placement of plugs to block the drainage of tears.

Due to LASIK eye surgery being a relatively new treatment option, long-term safety and effectiveness are unknown. The results of the procedure, however, may diminish with age and the natural changes that occur to the eye over time.

Q Are there other reasons besides LASIK to do laser eye surgery?

Yes, diabetic patients frequently require laser treatments to stabilize their eye condition (swelling in retina or new abnormal blood vessel growth on retina), glaucoma patients may require trabeculoplasty (lowers pressure by improving fluid outflow from eye) or iridotomy (hole made in iris of eye), and postoperative cataract patients frequently require capsulotomy procedures. These procedures are all done in office setting with topical eye drops for anesthesia.

Q How common is cataract surgery?

Cataract surgery is one of the most common eye surgeries. The majority of people who develop cataracts are usually older than 60 and their development can be regarded as part of the normal aging process in most cases. Other causes of cataracts include a history of trauma to the eye, side effects of certain drugs, exposure to toxic substances, medical conditions such as diabetes, and even by congenital means.

A cataract occurs when the natural lens of the eye, which is the part of the eye that helps us to focus on objects at different distances, becomes cloudy when it is normally transparent. Vision changes such as fuzziness, abnormal perception of colors, increased sensitivity to glare from light, distortion of your vision to seem as if you are looking through a veil, or even frequent changes in your eyeglasses prescription may occur.

Cataract surgery is almost always an elective surgery (meaning it is scheduled in advance) and very rarely an emergent one; therefore, if you are trying to decide whether to get cataract surgery consult your doctor for the options and timing which are best for you.

Q What is involved in cataract surgery?

Cataract surgery is the removal of the natural lens of the eye that has become cloudy, thereby distorting vision. In most cases a permanent artificial intraocular lens (IOL) replaces the removed lens to restore the eye's focusing ability.

The surgeon will use an operating microscope and make at least one small incision into the eye to remove the cataract, or the clouded lens. In this procedure the surgeon may use an ultrasound driven instrument that breaks up the cataract into sections which are then aspirated out. Another method your surgeon may use is to remove the cataract in one large piece that requires a larger incision.

In the next step of the operations your doctor will insert an artificial lens to replace the natural lens that was just removed.

Under most conditions the incisions made by your surgeon for cataract surgeries are self-healing. If a stitch is required to close the incision, your doctor will inform you if and when the stitch will need to be removed.

Q   After my eye surgery when can I continue with my normal activity?

Returning to normal activity after eye surgery depends on both what procedure you underwent as well as what your normal activity consists of. It is generally suggested to refrain from heavy lifting, bending, straining, and drinking until your post-operative visit. Returning to work also depends on what type of work you do. If you have a desk job, returning to work after a day of rest is usually acceptable. However, if your job involves strenuous activity, the risk of trauma to the eye, or the risk of wound contamination, it is suggested that you take a longer recovery period to prevent the risk of complications. If you are unsure of what activities you can resume contact your doctor for further instruction and advice.

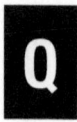 **My eyelids are droopy. In addition to the cosmetic effects will an eye lift help me see better?**

Through the common aging process the skin gradually loses its elasticity. This, with the effect of gravity, cause excessive skin to collect causing wrinkling of the lower lid and bulging of the upper lid which may form skin folds that can obstruct vision.

A surgical procedure called a blepharoplasty is used to remove the excess skin from the upper eyelid and to reduce the bagginess from the lower lid. The surgeon removes the excess skin, underlying fatty tissue, and muscle that caused the obstruction of the person's vision. Although the procedure is effective it will not stop the natural aging process.

Q | If I have glaucoma, how do I know if I need surgery?

Most cases of glaucoma are treated successfully with eye drops and rarely pills. However, when medications fail to treat glaucoma or you have an acute glaucoma attack laser or traditional surgery may be the best option.

Glaucoma is an eye condition caused by an increase in the pressure of the fluid in the front part of the eye. As this intraocular pressure increases it can cause damage to the optic nerve, the nerve which is responsible for transmitting the images from the eye to the brain. Permanent blindness can result from this condition without treatment.

There are several types of glaucoma with differences in both onset and presentation. The two main types are open-angle and closed-angle glaucoma. With closed-angle glaucoma there can be a sudden rise in intraocular pressure which may be associated with severe eye pain and redness of the eye, blurred vision, headache, nausea, and vomiting. This may result when the filtering angle (the drainage system called the trabecular meshwork located at the peripheral edge of the iris) is suddenly blocked.

In open-angle glaucoma, most people do not realize they have the condition until they begin to lose their vision because of the lack of symptoms. The gradual increases in pressure cause a continuing reduction of peripheral vision, called tunnel vision in its late stages. The exact cause of open-angle glaucoma is unknown but the condition tends to run in families and is particularly high risk in people of African descent.

An acute attack of glaucoma is considered a medical emergency and, in many cases, is relieved by eye surgery where the surgeon performs a laser iridotomy. The procedure involves making a small hole in the iris, the colored part of the eye, with a laser to resume the normal drainage of fluid.

Other surgeries to treat glaucoma include laser surgery called trabeculoplasty, a filtering surgery called trabeculectomy, and the placement of drainage implants. The trabeculoplasty surgery involves directing a laser beam at the clogged drainage channels in order open the canals and allow more fluid to drain. In a trabeculectomy the surgeon with remove a small piece of the trabecular meshwork allowing the fluid to freely leave the eye through this intraocular hole. Another treatment option is the placement of a drainage implant, which is a small tube precisely placed also to aid in the drainage of the fluid.

INTERVENTIONAL RADIOLOGY

// See Disclaimer on page 1 of this book before reading this chapter.

Authors:

SONIA VARMA, MS-III
St. George's University School of Medicine

Editors:

ERNEST WIGGINS, M.D.
Attending Physician, Interventional Radiology
Monmouth Medical Center, Long Branch, NJ

PASQUALE D. EVANGELISTA, M.D.
Resident Physician, Diagnostic and Interventional
Radiology Residency Training Program
Monmouth Medical Center, Long Branch, NJ

What is interventional radiology? How is it different from surgery?

Radiology is the branch of medicine that uses x-rays, CAT scans and ultrasound to look at the body. Interventional radiology (IR) is when the images of the body are used to deliver treatment to the patient. It is not the same as going in for surgery for a few reasons. Firstly, most IR procedures are performed in a special IR room of the hospital, not in the operating room (OR). That room has machines built in so that the images can be taken all throughout the procedure. The main difference between IR and general surgery is that in IR, the doctor can use the images to see inside the body without making a large incision. This is beneficial because it means that the procedure is minimally invasive - the doctor will only make small breaks in the skin at the important areas. Another benefit is that the patient is usually given a local numbing agent to the area, so they are not knocked out. This makes recovery time faster because the patient isn't groggy afterwards, and is usually able to go home right after. Overall, interventional radiology procedures are because the images help the doctor treat the patient faster and safer than traditional surgery methods.

Q   I have fibroids. Is getting a uterine fibroid embolization more effective than getting surgery? Do the results last forever?

Uterine fibroid embolization is an IR procedure that plugs up the blood supply to fibroids, causing them to shrink over time, compared to surgery, where an incision is made in the uterus and the fibroids are removed. The embolization technique is becoming increasingly popular over the years because it is a faster procedure and recovery is much better than fibroid removal by surgery. About 92% of women had their pain and bleeding symptoms improved after having the embolization done. This procedure may affect your ability to have children so you should discuss this with your doctor first. Many factors affect the success of this procedure, including the size of your fibroids. Your doctor will determine if fibroid embolization is right for you. As with all procedures, complications like infection are possible. As for the results of an embolization treatment, the existing fibroids shrink and new fibroids rarely appear. Overall, uterine fibroid embolization is a highly effective treatment with less pain and faster recovery, but it may not be for everyone.

The doctor is asking me about taking contrast for the procedure. Should I?

Taking contrast is when you drink a liquid or get an injection of a material, which lights up on imaging to show the doctor a roadmap of your blood vessels or your digestive system, depending on what you are being treated for. This shows the doctor where everything is, which guides him through the procedure and improves your care. Therefore, if you are being asked to take contrast for your procedure, it is recommended that you do take it. However, there are situations where taking contrast could cause problems for you. Any medications you are on could interfere with the contrast, so tell your doctor about what you are taking. Sometimes, patients have allergies to the contrast agent used, which can cause hives and wheezing. There can be worse allergic reactions than that, but they are less common. If you experience any allergic reaction, the IR health care team will give you Benedryl or epinephrine

which will help your symptoms. Besides allergies, contrast can affect the kidneys which can lead to kidney failure, which can be serious. This happens more in patients who already have kidney problems, which is something the IR department can check for by measuring your blood levels if you give your consent. Basically, contrast makes images of your body more clear so that the doctor can see more clearly inside your body, but it may cause adverse reactions so make sure you discuss with your doctor about allergies, medications and kidney problems you may have.

Q Are there any damaging effects from all the radiation I am receiving during my procedure?

There are 4 different types of imaging that doctors use in IR: x-ray, ultrasound, CAT scan and MRI. Some types involve no radiation at all, like ultrasound and MRI. However, x-ray and CAT scan do expose your body to radiation. The amount of radiation is very different between these two techniques – a CAT scan is a more sophisticated x-ray machine, and therefore it uses over 100 times more radiation on your body. Radiation to your body should be done only when it is absolutely necessary to benefit your health, and therefore it would outweigh the risks caused by irradiation. Also, the damage caused by radiation is different for each organ. Breast tissue is the most affected by radiation, which may increase the risk of breast cancer over time. This is a serious problem, so during a CAT scan women are usually given a metal plate to put on their chest to act as a breast shield – it reduces the radiation reaching that area. Speak to your doctor if you have a history of breast cancer in your family before getting images done. Other parts of the body, like the neck and groin area, may be covered by a lead apron to also protect against radiation damage. Radiation mostly affects people between the ages of 2 and 40 years old, so if your child is having an image taken, talk to the doctor about protecting them from too much radiation exposure at a young age.

In a typical IR procedure, the radiation to produce the images is controlled by a pedal on the floor that the doctor can press anytime he wants to got an image. The amount of radiation in your procedure is determined by the amount of time he is pressing on the pedal. If you have any concerns, talk to your doctor about how he is planning on using the pump and how many images will be made. Lastly, it is always good to keep a list of how many x-rays and CAT scans you have had done, and what part of the body they were imaging. Then you can take that list whenever you see your doctor about getting IR procedures or images taken. This is a good way of keeping track of how much radiation you have received for health care, and how it may affect your future care.

Q | How do I find a hospital with an IR doctor?

IR procedures cover many areas of health care, from doing biopsies and clearing clogged blood vessels, to fixing unsightly varicose veins. You may find that an IR procedure is available for your health care needs and is better suited to you than alternative methods, such as taking medication. If this is the case, you can find an accredited IR doctor by visiting the American College of Radiology website (www. acr.org) and filling in the type of imaging study you will be getting. Also, you can visit the website of the Society of Interventional Radiology (www.sirweb.org) to learn more about them, and about the procedure they will be performing on you. This can help you prepare for your procedure, and make you feel at ease about the sights and sounds that you will be experiencing in the IR room.

APPENDIX: CITATIONS

Chapter 1: Emergency Surgery

Abboud, H, Henrich, WL. Clinical practice. Stage IV chronic kidney disease. N Engl J Med 2010; 362:56.

Ansell, J, Hirsh, J, Hylek, E, et al. Pharmacology and management of the vitamin K antagonists: American College of Chest Physicians Evidence-Based Clinical Practice Guidelines (8th Edition). Chest 2008; 133:160S.

Aspelin, P, Aubry, P, Fransson, SG, et al. Nephrotoxic effects in high-risk patients undergoing angiography. N Engl J Med 2003; 348:491.

Berend, K, Levi, M. Management of adult Jehovah's Witness patients with acute bleeding. Am J Med 2009; 122:1071.

Bittner, RC, Felix, R. Magnetic resonance (MR) imaging of the chest: State-of-the-art. Eur Respir J 1998; 11:1392.

Contreras, G, Pardo, V, Cely, C. Factors associated with poor outcomes in patients with lupus nephritis. Lupus 2005; 14:890.

Costacou, T, Ellis, D, Fried, L, Orchard, TJ. Sequence of progression of albuminuria and decreased GFR in persons with type 1 diabetes: a cohort study. Am J Kidney Dis 2007; 50:721.

Crowe, SE, Perdue, MH. Gastrointestinal food hypersensitivity: basic mechanisms of pathophysiology. Gastroenterology 1992; 103:1075.

Cuende, N, Miranda, B, Canon, JF, et al. Donor characteristics associated with liver graft survival. Transplantation 2005; 79:1445.

Elliott, KG, Johnstone, AJ. Diagnosing acute compartment syndrome. J Bone Joint Surg Br 2003; 85:625.

Fishman, JA. Infection in solid-organ transplant recipients. N Engl J Med 2007; 357:2601.

Glotz, D, Antoine, C, Duboust, A. Antidonor antibodies and transplantation: How to deal with them before and after transplantation. Transplantation 2005; 79:S30.

Harmening, DM. Modern blood banking and transfusion practices, 5th ed, F.A. Davis Company, Philadelphia 2005.

Henderson, R, Jabbour, N, Zeger, G. Legal and administrative issues relate to transfusion-free medicine and surgery. In: Transfusion-free medicine and surgery, Jabbor, N (Ed), Blackwell, Malden, MA 2005. p.1.

Igarashi, P, Somlo, S. Genetics and pathogenesis of polycystic kidney disease. J Am Soc Nephrol 2002; 13:2384.

Jaffe, BM, Berger, DH. The Appendix. In: Schwartz Principles of Surgery, 8th ed, Schwartz, SI, Brunicardi, CF (Ed), McGraw-Hill Health Pub. Division, New York 2005.

Kwok, MY, Kim, MK, Gorelick, MH. Evidence-based approach to the diagnosis of appendicitis in children. Pediatr Emerg Care 2004; 20:690.

Lieberman, P, Camargo, CA, Jr, Bohlke, K, et al. Epidemiology of anaphylaxis: findings of the American College of Allergy, Asthma and Immunology Epidemiology of Anaphylaxis Working Group. Ann Allergy Asthma Immunol 2006; 97:596.

Ljung, RC. Intracranial haemorrhage in haemophilia A and B. Br J Haematol 2008; 140:378. Mackenzie, CF, Morrison, C, Jaberi, M, et al. Management of hemorrhagic shock when blood is not an option. J Clin Anesth 2008; 20:538.

Meisel, A, Snyder, L, Quill, T. Seven legal barriers to end-of-life care: myths, realities, and grains of truth. The American College of Physician-American Society of Internal Medicine End-of-Life Care Consensus Panel. JAMA 2000; 284:2495.

MRI safety. Institute for Magnetic Resonance Safety, Education, and Research Web site. Available at: http://222.MRIsafety.com. Accessed August 6, 2010.

Nakamura, T, Fukuda, K, Hayakawa, K, et al. Mechanism of burn injury during magnetic resonance imaging (MRI)--simple loops can induce heat injury. Front Med Biol Eng 2001; 11:117.

Nash, MJ, Cohen, H. Management of Jehovah's Witness patients with haematological problems. Blood Rev 2004; 18:211.

Ong, AC, Harris, PC. Molecular pathogenesis of ADPKD: The polycystin complex gets complex. Kidney Int 2005; 67:1234.

Office of the Chief Medical Examiner – Frequently Asked Questions. http://home2.nyc. gov/html/ocme/html/faq/faq.shtml. Accessed August 7, 2010.

Oswalt, ML, Kemp, SF. Anaphylaxis: office management and prevention. Immunol Allergy Clin North Am 2007; 27:177.

Rizvi, S, Catenacci, M. Responding promptly to acute compartment syndrome. Emerg Med 2008; 40:12.

Rothrock, SG, Pagane, J. Acute appendicitis in children: emergency department diagnosis and management. Ann Emerg Med 2000; 36:39.

Thromb Haemost 2001; 85:560. Chung, CH, Ng, CP, Lai, KK. Delays by patients, emergency physicians, and surgeons in the management of acute appendicitis: retrospective study. Hong Kong Med J 2000; 6:254.

Tormey, CA, Stack, G. The persistence and evanescence of blood group alloantibodies in men. Transfusion 2009; 49:505.

Tosetto, A, Castaman, G, Rodeghiero, F. Evidence-based diagnosis of type 1 von Willebrand disease: a Bayes theorem approach. Blood 2008; 111:3998.

Sadler, JE, Mannucci, PM, Berntorp, E, et al. Impact, diagnosis and treatment of von Willebrand disease. Thromb Haemost 2000; 84:160.

Sampson, HA. Anaphylaxis and emergency treatment. Pediatrics 2003; 111:1601. Schulman, S. Care of patients receiving long-term anticoagulant therapy. N Engl J Med 2003; 349:675

Shalowitz, DI, Garrett-Mayer, E, Wendler, D. The accuracy of surrogate decision makers: a systematic review. Arch Intern Med 2006; 166:493.

Steinman, TI, Becker, BN, Frost, AE, et al. Guidelines for the referral and management of patients eligible for solid organ transplantation. Transplantation 2001; 71:1189.

Shirani, J, Pick, R, Roberts, WC, Maron, BJ. Morphology and significance of the left ventricular collagen network in young patients with hypertrophic cardiomyopathy and sudden cardiac death. J Am Coll Cardiol 2000; 35:36.

Sokol, RJ, Hewitt, S, Booker, DJ, Morris, BM. Patients with red cell autoantibodies: Selection of blood for transfusion. Clin Lab Haematol 1988; 10:257.

Storaas, T, Steinsvag, SK, Florvaag, E, et al. Occupational rhinitis: diagnostic criteria, relation to lower airway symptoms and IgE sensitization in bakery workers. Acta Otolaryngol 2005; 125:1211.

Thong, BY, Yeow-Chan, . Anaphylaxis during surgical and interventional procedures. Ann Allergy Asthma Immunol 2004; 92:619.

Vamvakas, EC, Blajchman, MA. Transfusion-related mortality: the ongoing risks of allogeneic blood transfusion and the available strategies for their prevention. Blood 2009; 113:3406.

Weisbord, SD, Palevsky, PM. Radiocontrast-induced acute renal failure. J Intensive Care Med 2005; 20:63.

White, GC 2nd, Rosendaal, F, Aledort, LM, et al. Definitions in hemophilia. Recommendation of the scientific subcommittee on factor VIII and factor IX of the scientific and standardization committee of the International Society on Thrombosis and Haemostasis. Factor VII and Factor IX Subcommittee.

Chapter 2: Internal & Perioperative Medicine

Blumenfeld YJ, Wong AE, Jafari A, Barth RA, El-Sayed YY. MR imaging in cases of antenatal suspected appendicitis - a meta-analysis. J Matern Fetal Neonatal Med. ePub 2010 Aug 9.

Butala P, Greenstein AJ, Sur MD, Mehta N, Sadot E, Divino CM. Surgical Management of Acute Right Lower-Quadrant Pain in Pregnancy: A Prospective Cohort Study. J Am Coll Surg. ePub 2010 Aug 6.

Caruso GA, Capodanno D, Giannone MT, Giannazzo D, Monte I, Nigro P, Sorrentino F.The usefulness of clinical indexes in the evaluation of cardiovascular risk in non cardiac surgery. Minerva Cardioangiol. 2006 Dec;54(6):763-72.

Cochrane Database Syst Rev. 2010 Jul 7;7:CD001484. Elastic compression stockings for prevention of deep vein thrombosis. Sachdeva A, Dalton M, Amaragiri SV, Lees T.

Colman-Brochu S. Deep vein thrombosis in pregnancy. MCN Am J Matern Child Nurs. 2004 May-Jun;29(3):186-92.

Dionigi R, Dionigi G, Rovera F, Boni L. Postoperative fever. Surg Infect (Larchmt). 2006;7 Suppl 2:S17-20.

Gleckman RA, Roth RM. Fever following abdominal surgery. Unusual infectious causes. Postgrad Med. 1986 Feb 1;79(2):287-94.

Hedenstierna G, Edmark L. Mechanisms of atelectasis in the perioperative period. Best Pract Res Clin Anaesthesiol. 2010 Jun;24(2):157-69.

Lehot JJ, Arvieux CC, Viale JP, Foëx P. Myocardial ischemia and anesthesia. Ann Fr Anesth Reanim. 1995;14(2):176-97.

Makar GA, Ginsberg GG. Therapy insight: approaching endoscopy in anticoagulated patients. Nat Clin Pract Gastroenterol Hepatol. 2006 Jan;3(1):43-52.

Normal ranges for common laboratory test. http://www.rush.edu/webapps/rml/RMLRanges.jsp. Accessed September 8, 2010.

Perioperative Anticoagulation Management. http://emedicine.medscape.com/article/285265-overview. Accessed September 6, 2010.

Rinfret S, Goldman L, Polanczyk CA, Cook EF, Lee TH. Value of immediate postoperative electrocardiogram to update risk stratification after major noncardiac surgery. Am J Cardiol. 2004 Oct 15;94(8):1017-22.

Rowe DJ, Baker AC. Perioperative risks and benefits of herbal supplements in aesthetic surgery. Aesthet Surg J. 2009 Mar-Apr;29(2):150-7.

Vernick W, Fleisher LA. Risk stratification. Best Pract Res Clin Anaesthesiol. 2008 Mar;22(1):1-21.

What You Should Know About Herbal and Dietary Supplement Use and Anesthesia. http://www.asahq.org/patientEducation/herbPatient.pdf. Accessed September 7, 2010

Williams PM, Fletcher S. Health effects of prenatal radiation exposure. Am Fam Physician. 2010 Sep 1;82(5):488-93.

Chapter 3: Anesthesiology & Pain Management

2005 American Heart Association Guidelines for Cardiopulmonary Resuscitation and Emergency Cardiovascular Care. Circulation 2005; 112:IV1.

2005 American Heart Association (AHA) guidelines for cardiopulmonary resuscitation

(CPR) and emergency cardiovascular care (ECC) of pediatric and neonatal patients: neonatal resuscitation guidelines. Pediatrics 2006; 117:e1029.

2005 International Consensus on Cardiopulmonary Resuscitation and Emergency Cardiovascular Care Science with Treatment Recommendations. Part 2: Adult basic life support. Resuscitation 2005; 67:187.

Abella, BS, Sandbo, N, Vassilatos, P, et al. Chest compression rates during cardiopulmonary resuscitation are suboptimal: a prospective study during in-hospital cardiac arrest. Circulation 2005; 111:428.

Balsells, F, Wyllie, R, Kay, M, Steffen, R. Use of conscious sedation for lower and upper gastrointestinal endoscopic examinations in children, adolescents, and young adults: A twelve-year review. Gastrointest Endosc 1997; 45:375.

Bower, AL, Ripepi, A, Dilger, J, et al. Bispectral index monitoring of sedation during endoscopy. Gastrointest Endosc 2000; 52:192.

Brady, JE, Sun, LS, Rosenberg, H, Li, G. Prevalence of malignant hyperthermia due to anesthesia in New York State, 2001-2005. Anesth Analg 2009; 109:1162.

Chaudhri, BB, Macfie, A, Kirk, AJ. Inadvertent total spinal anesthesia after intercostal nerve block placement during lung resection. Ann Thorac Surg 2009; 88:283.

Coveney, E, Weltz, CR, Greengrass, R, et al. Use of paravertebral block anesthesia in the surgical management of breast cancer: experience in 156 cases. Ann Surg 1998; 227:496.

Denborough, M. Malignant hyperthermia. Lancet 1998; 352:1131.

Eichenberger, U, Greher, M, Kirchmair, L, et al. Ultrasound-guided blocks of the ilioinguinal and iliohypogastric nerve: accuracy of a selective new technique confirmed by anatomical dissection. Br J Anaesth 2006; 97:238.

de Beer, Jde V, Winemaker, MJ, Donnelly, GA, et al. Efficacy and safety of controlled-release oxycodone and standard therapies for postoperative pain after knee or hip replacement. Can J Surg 2005; 48:277.

Deakin, CD, Nolan, JP, European Resuscitation, C. European Resuscitation Council guidelines for resuscitation 2005. Section 3. Electrical therapies: automated external defibrillators, defibrillation, cardioversion and pacing. Resuscitation 2005; 67 Suppl 1;S25.

Denborough, MA, Forster, JF, Lovell, RR, et al. Anaesthetic deaths in a family. Br J Anaesth 1962; 34:395.

Devereaux, PJ, Goldman, L, Cook, DJ, et al. Perioperative cardiac events in patients undergoing noncardiac surgery: a review of the magnitude of the problem, the pathophysiology of the events and methods to estimate and communicate risk. CMAJ 2005; 173:627.

Dirks, J, Fredensborg, BB, Christensen, D, et al. A randomized study of the effects of single-dose gabapentin versus placebo on postoperative pain and morphine consumption after mastectomy. Anesthesiology 2002; 97:560.

Faigel, DO, Baron, TH, Goldstein, JL, et al. Guidelines for the use of deep sedation and anesthesia for GI endoscopy. Gastrointest Endosc 2002; 56:613.

Fleisher, LA, Beckman, JA, Brown, KA, et al. ACC/AHA 2007 guidelines on perioperative cardiovascular evaluation and care for noncardiac surgery: a report of the American College of Cardiology/American Heart Association Task Force on Practice Guidelines (Writing Committee to Revise the 2002 Guidelines on Perioperative Cardiovascular Evaluation for Noncardiac Surgery) developed in collaboration with the American Society of Echocardiography, American Society of Nuclear Cardiology, Heart Rhythm Society, Society of Cardiovascular Anesthesiologists, Society for Cardiovascular Angiography and Interventions, Society for Vascular Medicine and Biology, and Society for Vascular Surgery. J Am Coll Cardiol 2007; 50:e159.

Fleisher, LA, Pasternak, LR, Herbert, R, Anderson, GF. Inpatient hospital admission and death after outpatient surgery in elderly patients: importance of patient and system characteristics and location of care. Arch Surg 2004; 139:67.

Jorgensen, H, Wetterslev, J, Moiniche, S, Dahl, JB. Epidural local anaesthetics versus opioid-based analgesic regimens on postoperative gastrointestinal paralysis, PONV and pain after abdominal surgery. Cochrane Database Syst Rev 2000

Karmakar, MK, Ho, AMH. Acute pain management of patients with multiple fractured ribs. J Trauma 2003; 54:615.

Larach, MG, Gronert, GA, Allen, GC, et al. Clinical presentation, treatment, and complications of malignant hyperthermia in North America from 1987 to 2006. Anesth Analg 2010; 110:498.

Lindenauer, PK, Pekow, P, Wang, K, et al. Perioperative beta-blocker therapy and mortality after major noncardiac surgery. N Engl J Med 2005; 353:349.

Maurer, SG, Chen, AL, Hiebert, R, et al. Comparison of outcomes of using spinal versus general anesthesia in total hip arthroplasty. Am J Orthop 2007; 36:E101.

Mixter, CG 3rd, Meeker, LD, Gavin, TJ. Preemptive pain control in patients having laparoscopic hernia repair: a comparison of keterolac and ibuprofen. Arch Surg 1998;133:432.

Ong, CK, Lirk, P, Seymour, RA, Jenkins, BJ. The efficacy of preemptive analgesia for acute postoperative pain management: a meta-analysis. Anesth Analg 2005; 100:757.

Pandit, JJ, Satya-Krishna, R, Gration, P. Superficial or deep cervical plexus block for carotid endarterectomy: a systematic review of complications. Br J Anaesth 2007; 99:159.

Pandey, CK, Priye, S, Singh, S, et al. Preemptive use of gabapentin significantly decreases postoperative pain and rescue analgesic requirements in laparoscopic cholecystectomy. Can J Anaesth 2004; 51:358.

Poirier, P, Alpert, MA, Fleisher, LA, et al. Cardiovascular evaluation and management of severely obese patients undergoing surgery: a science advisory from the American Heart Association. Circulation 2009; 120:86.

Polanczyk, CA, et al. Right heart catheterization and cardiac complications in patients undergoing noncardiac surgery: an observational study. JAMA 2001; 286:309.

Pollard, RJ, Coyle, JP, Gilbert, RL, Beck, JE. Intraoperative awareness in a regional medical system: a review of 3 years' data. Anesthesiology 2007; 106:269.

Ranta, SO, Laurila, R, Saario, J, et al. Awareness with recall during general anesthesia: incidence and risk factors. Anesth Analg 1998; 86:1084.

Rodseth, RN, Padayachee, L, Biccard, BM. A meta-analysis of the utility of pre-operative brain natriuretic peptide in predicting early and intermediate-term mortality and major adverse cardiac events in vascular surgical patients. Anaesthesia 2008; 63:1226.

Rose, DK, Cohen, MM. The airway: problems and predictions in 18,500 patients. Can J Anaesth 1994; 41:372.

Rosenberg, H, Davis, M, James, D, et al. Malignant hyperthermia. Orphanet J Rare Dis 2007; 2:21.

Rungreungvanich, M, Thienthong, S, Charuluxananan, S, et al. Predictors of intra-operative recall of awareness: Thai Anesthesia Incidents Study (THAI Study): a case-control study. J Med Assoc Thai 2007; 90:1551.

Sanders, RD, Weimann, J, Maze, M. Biologic effects of nitrous oxide: a mechanistic and toxicologic review. Anesthesiology 2008; 109:707.

Scott, DA, Blake, D, Buckland, M, et al. A comparison of epidural ropivacaine infusion alone and in combination with 1, 2, and 4 microg/mL fentanyl for seventy-two hours of postoperative analgesia after major abdominal surgery. Anesth Analg 1999; 88:857.

Scott, DB, Lee, A, Fagan, D, et al. Acute toxicity of ropivacaine compared with that of bupivacaine. Anesth Analg 1989; 69:563.

Senard, M, Joris, JL, Ledoux, D, et al. A comparison of 0.1% and 0.2% ropivacaine and bupivacaine combined with morphine for postoperative patient-controlled epidural analgesia after major abdominal surgery. Anesth Analg 2002; 95:444.

Singh, H, Poluha, W, Cheung, M, et al. Propofol for sedation during colonoscopy. Cochrane Database Syst Rev 2008; (4).

Ulmer, BJ, Hansen, JJ, Overley, CA, et al. Propofol versus midazolam/fentanyl for outpatient colonoscopy: administration by nurses supervised by endoscopists. Clin Gastroenterol Hepatol 2003; 1:425.

Watcha, MF, Issioui, T, Klein, KW, White, PF. Costs and effectiveness of rofecoxib, celecoxib, and acetaminophen for preventing pain after ambulatory otolaryngologic surgery. Anesth Analg 2003; 96:987.

White, PF, Kehlet, H, Neal, JM, et al. The role of the anesthesiologist in fast-track surgery: from multimodal analgesia to perioperative medical care. Anesth Analg 2007; 104:1380.

Wilcox, CM, Linder, J. Prospective evaluation of droperidol on sphincter of oddi motility. Gastrointest Endosc 2003; 58:483.

Chapter 4: General Surgery

Ananda, SS, McLaughlin, SJ, Chen, F. Initial impact of Australia's National Bowel Cancer Screening Program. Med J Aust 2009; 191:378.

Baker, JB, Mandavia, D, Swadron, SP. Diagnosis of diverticulitis by bedside ultrasound in the Emergency Department. J Emerg Med 2006; 30:327.

Borrelli, O, Cordischi, L, Cirulli, M. Polymeric diet alone versus corticosteroids in the treatment of active pediatric Crohn's disease: a randomized controlled open-label trial. Clin Gastroenterol Hepatol 2006; 4:744.

Cales, P, Masliah, C, Bernard, B. Early administration of vapreotide for variceal bleeding in patients with cirrhosis. N Engl J Med 2001; 344:23.

Cardenas, A, Uriz, J, Gines, P, Arroyo, V. Hepatorenal syndrome. Liver Transpl 2000; 6:S63.

Cardillo, G, Carleo, F, Carbone, L. Long-term lung function following videothoracoscopic talc poudrage for primary spontaneous recurrent pneumothorax. Eur J Cardiothorac Surg 2007; 31:802.

DeVault, KR, Castell, DO; American College of Gastroenterology. Updated guidelines for the diagnosis and treatment of gastroesophageal reflux disease. Am J Gastroenterol 2005; 100:190.

Diehl, AK. Gallstone size and the risk of gallbladder cancer. JAMA 1983; 250:2323.

Goh, V, Halligan, S, Taylor, SA. Differentiation between diverticulitis and colorectal cancer: quantitative CT perfusion measurements versus morphologic criteria--initial experience. Radiology 2007; 242:456.

Gunderson, LL, Jessup, JM, Sargent, DJ. Revised TN categorization for colon cancer based on national survival outcomes data. J Clin Oncol 2010; 28:264.

Gunderson, LL, Jessup, JM, Sargent, DJ. Revised tumor and node categorization for rectal cancer based on surveillance, epidemiology, and end results and rectal pooled analysis outcomes. J Clin Oncol 2010; 28:256.

Hadengue, A, Benhayoun, MK, Lebrec, D, Benhamou, JP. Pulmonary hypertension complicating portal hypertension: prevalence and relation to splanchnic hemodynamics. Gastroenterology 1991; 100:520.

Hunt, I, Barber, B, Southon, R, Treasure, T. Is talc pleurodesis safe for young patients following primary spontaneous pneumothorax?. Interact Cardiovasc Thorac Surg 2007; 6:117.

Kalyanasundaram, A, Elmore, JR, Manazer, JR. Simvastatin suppresses experimental aortic aneurysm expansion. J Vasc Surg 2006; 43:117.

Memon, MA, Cooper, NJ, Memon, B. Meta-analysis of randomized clinical trials comparing open and laparoscopic inguinal hernia repair. Br J Surg 2003; 90:1479.

Neumayer, L, Giobbie-Hurder, A, Jonasson, O. Open mesh versus laparoscopic mesh repair of inguinal hernia. N Engl J Med 2004; 350:1819.

Propranolol for small abdominal aortic aneurysms: results of a randomized trial. J Vasc Surg 2002; 35:72.

Shiffman, ML, Sugerman, HJ, Kellum, JM. Gallstone formation after rapid weight loss: a prospective study in patients undergoing gastric bypass surgery for treatment of morbid obesity. Am J Gastroenterol 1991; 86:1000.

Uhlen, S, Belbouab, R, Narebski, K. Efficacy of methotrexate in pediatric Crohn's disease: a French multicenter study. Inflamm Bowel Dis 2006; 12:1053.

Yang, YX., Lewis, JD, Epstein, S, Metz, DC. Long-term proton pump inhibitor therapy and risk of hip fracture. JAMA 2006; 296:2947.

Chapter 5: Thoracic Surgery: Heart, Lungs, & Esophagus

Alexander, KP, Newby, LK, Armstrong, PW. Acute coronary care in the elderly, part II: ST-segment-elevation myocardial infarction: a scientific statement for healthcare professionals from the American Heart Association Council on Clinical Cardiology: in collaboration with the Society of Geriatric Cardiology. Circulation 2007; 115:2570.

Alpert, JS, Thygesen, K, Antman, E, Bassand, JP. Myocardial infarction redefined--a consensus document of The Joint European Society of Cardiology/American College of Cardiology Committee for the redefinition of myocardial infarction. J Am Coll Cardiol 2000; 36:959.

Anderson, J, Adams, C, Antman, E. ACC/AHA 2007 guidelines for the management of patients with unstable angina/non-ST-elevation myocardial infarction: a report of the American College of Cardiology/American Heart Association Task Force on Practice Guidelines (Writing Committee to revise the 2002 Guidelines for the Management of Patients with Unstable Angina/Non-ST-Elevation Myocardial Infarction): developed in collaboration with the American College of Emergency Physicians, American College or Physicians, Society for Academic Emergency Medicine, Society for Cardiovascular

Angiography and Interventions, and Society of Thoracic Surgeons. J Am Coll Cardiol 2007; 50:e1. Available at: www.acc.org/qualityandscience/clinical/statements.htm. Accessed July 18, 2010.

American Academy of Pediatrics, American College of Obstetricians and Gynecologists; Guidelines for Perinatal Care, 6th Ed, American Academy of Pediatrics, Elk Grove Village, IL 2008.

Balady, GJ, Williams, MA, Ades, PA. Core components of cardiac rehabilitation/secondary prevention programs: 2007 update: a scientific statement from the American Heart Association Exercise, Cardiac Rehabilitation, and Prevention Committee, the Council on Clinical Cardiology; the Councils on Cardiovascular Nursing, Epidemiology and Prevention, and Nutrition, Physical Activity, and Metabolism; and the American Association of Cardiovascular and Pulmonary Rehabilitation. Circulation 2007; 115:2675.

Bassan, R, Pimenta, L, Scofano, M. Probability stratification and systematic diagnostic approach for chest pain patients in the emergency department. Crit Pathw Cardiol 2004; 3:1.

Bonow, RO, Carabello, BA, Chatterjee, K. 2008 Focused update incorporated into the ACC/AHA 2006 guidelines for the management of patients with valvular heart disease: a report of the American College of Cardiology/American Heart Association Task Force on Practice Guidelines (Writing Committee to Revise the 1998 Guidelines for the Management of Patients With Valvular Heart Disease): endorsed by the Society of Cardiovascular Anesthesiologists, Society for Cardiovascular Angiography and Interventions, and Society of Thoracic Surgeons. Circulation 2008; 118:e523.

Cannegieter, SC, Rosendaal, FR, Wintzen, AR. Optimal oral anticoagulant therapy in patients with mechanical heart valves. N Engl J Med 1995; 333:11.

Cardiac Rehabilitation, and Prevention) and the Council on Nutrition, Physical Activity, and Metabolism (Subcommittee on Physical Activity), in Collaboration with the American Association of Cardiovascular and Pulmonary Rehabilitation. Circulation 2005; 111:369.Clark, AM, Hartling, L, Vandermeer, B, McAlister, FA. Meta-analysis: secondary prevention programs for patients with coronary artery disease. Ann Intern Med 2005; 143:659.

Cleveland, JC Jr, Shroyer, AL, Chen, AY. Off-pump coronary artery bypass grafting decreases risk-adjusted mortality and morbidity. Ann Thorac Surg 2001; 72:1282.

Douketis, JD, Berger, PB, Dunn, AS. The perioperative management of antithrombotic therapy: American College of Chest Physicians Evidence-Based Clinical Practice Guidelines (8th Edition). Chest 2008; 133:299S.

Fesmire, FM, Percy, RF, Bardoner, JB. Usefulness of automated serial 12-lead ECG monitoring during the initial emergency department evaluation of patients with chest pain. Ann Emerg Med 1998; 31:3.

Freeman, RV, Otto, CM. Spectrum of calcific aortic valve disease: pathogenesis, disease progression, and treatment strategies. Circulation 2005; 111:3316.

Harrington, RA, Becker, RC, Cannon, CP. Antithrombotic therapy for non-ST-segment elevation acute coronary syndromes: American College of Chest Physicians Evidence-Based Clinical Practice Guidelines (8th Edition). Chest 2008; 133:670S.

Jaffe, AS, Babuin, L, Apple, FS. Biomarkers in acute cardiac disease: the present and the future. J Am Coll Cardiol 2006; 48:1.

Kontozis, L, Skudicky, D, Hopley, MJ. Long-term follow-up of St. Jude medical prosthesis in a young rheumatic population using low-level warfarin anticoagulation: An analysis of the temporal distribution of cause of death. Am J Cardiol 1998; 81:736.

Kushner, FG, Hand, M, Smith, SC Jr. 2009 Focused Updates: ACC/AHA Guidelines for the Management of Patients With ST-Elevation Myocardial Infarction (updating the 2004 Guideline and 2007 Focused Update) and ACC/AHA/SCAI Guidelines on Percutaneous Coronary Intervention (updating the 2005 Guideline and 2007 Focused Update): a report of the American College of Cardiology Foundation/American Heart Association Task Force on Practice Guidelines. Circulation 2009; 120:2271. Available at:http://circ.ahajournals.org/cgi/reprint/CIRCULATIONAHA.109.192663. Accessed July 16, 2010.

Kooley, EC, Roura, JA, Grines, CL. Primary angioplasty versus intravenous thrombolytic therapy for acute myocardial infarction. a quantitative review of 23 randomised trials. Lancet 2003; 361:13.

Larson, RJ, Fisher, ES. Should aspirin be continued in patients started on warfarin?. J Gen Intern Med 2004; 19:879.

Leon, AS, Franklin, BA, Costa, F. Cardiac rehabilitation and secondary prevention of coronary heart disease. An American Heart Association Scientific Statement from the Council on Clinical Cardiology (Subcommittee on Exercise,

Lissauer, T. Physical examination of the newborn. In: Neonatal-Perinatal Medicine:

Diseases of the Fetus and Infant, 8th ed, Fanaroff, AA, Martin, RJ, Walsh, MC, (Eds), Mosby, St Louis, 2006, p. 513.

Lopez-Sendon, J, Swedberg, K, McMurray, J. Expert consensus document on beta-adrenergic receptor blockers. Eur Heart J 2004; 25:1341.

Mehta, RH, Rathore, SS, Radford, MJ. Acute myocardial infarction in the elderly: differences by age. J Am Coll Cardiol 2001; 38:736.

Morrow, DA, Antman, EM, Parsons, L. Application of the TIMI risk score for ST-elevation MI in the National Registry of Myocardial Infarction 3. JAMA 2001; 286:1356.

Otto, CM. Valvular aortic stenosis: disease severity and timing of intervention. J Am Coll Cardiol 2006; 47:2141.

Roberts, WC, Ko, JM. Frequency by decades of unicuspid, bicuspid, and tricuspid aortic valves in adults having isolated aortic valve replacement for aortic stenosis, with or without associated aortic regurgitation. Circulation 2005; 111:920.

Tanner, K, Sabrine, N, Wren, C. Cardiovascular malformations among preterm infants. Pediatrics 2005; 116:e833.

Thompson, PD, Franklin, BA, Balady, GJ. Exercise and acute cardiovascular events placing the risks into perspective: a scientific statement from the American Heart Association Council on Nutrition, Physical Activity, and Metabolism and the Council on Clinical Cardiology. Circulation 2007; 115:2358.

Thygesen, K, Alpert, JS, White, HD. Universal definition of myocardial infarction: Kristian Thygesen, Joseph S. Alpert and Harvey D. White on behalf of the Joint ESC/ACCF/AHA/WHF Task Force for the Redefinition of Myocardial Infarction. Eur Heart J 2007; 28:2525.

Vahanian, A, Baumgartner, H, Bax, J. Guidelines on the management of valvular heart disease: The Task Force on the Management of Valvular Heart Disease of the European Society of Cardiology. Eur Heart J 2007; 28:230.

Vongpatanasin, W, Hillis, LD, Lange, RA. Prosthetic heart valves. N Engl J Med 1996; 335:407.

Wren, C, Reinhardt, Z, Khawaja, K. Twenty-year trends in diagnosis of life-threatening neonatal cardiovascular malformations. Arch Dis Child Fetal Neonatal Ed 2008; 93:F33.

Chapter 6: Orthopedic Surgery: Bones, Limbs, & Muscles

Albright, JC, Carpenter, JE, Graf, BK. Knee and leg: soft tissue trauma. In: Orthopaedic Knowledge Update 6, Beaty, JH, (Ed), American Academy of Orthopaedic Surgeons, Rosemont IL 1999. p.533.

Alfredson, H, Lorentzon, R. Chronic achilles tendinosis: recommendations for treatment and prevention. Sports Med 2000; 29:135.

Anderson, BC. Office Orthopedics for Primary Care: Diagnosis and Treatment, 3rd ed, Elsevier Saunders Company, Philadelphia, 2006.

Baek, GH, Kim, JH, Chung, MS. The natural history of pediatric trigger thumb. J Bone Joint Surg Am 2008; 90:980.

Beeres, FJ, Rhemrev, SJ, den Hollander, P. Early magnetic resonance imaging compared with bone scintigraphy in suspected scaphoid fractures. J Bone Joint Surg Br 2008; 90:1205.

Bhat, M, McCarthy, M, Davis, TR. MRI and plain radiography in the assessment of displaced fractures of the waist of the carpal scaphoid. J Bone Joint Surg Br 2004; 86:705.

Bisset, L, Beller, E, Jull, G. Mobilisation with movement and exercise, corticosteroid injection, or wait and see for tennis elbow: randomised trial. BMJ 2006; 333:939.

Breederveld, RS, Tuinebreijer, WE. Investigation of computed tomographic scan concurrent criterion validity in doubtful scaphoid fracture of the wrist. J Trauma 2004; 57:851.

Carson, S, Woolridge, DP, Colletti, J, Kilgore, K. Pediatric upper extremity injuries. Pediatr Clin North Am 2006; 53:41.

Chamberlain, JM, Patel, KM, Pollack, MM. Recalibration of the pediatric risk of admission score using a multi-institutional sample. Ann Emerg Med 2004; 43:461.

Colbourn, J, Heath, N, Manary, S, Pacifico, D. Effectiveness of splinting for the treatment of trigger finger. J Hand Ther 2008; 21:336.

Crowther, JD, Lachiewicz, PF. Survival and polyethylene wear of porous-coated acetabular components in patients less than fifty years old: results at nine to fourteen years. J Bone Joint Surg Am 2002; 84-A:729.

DeHart, MM, Riley, LH Jr. Nerve injuries in total hip arthroplasty. J Am Acad Orthop Surg 1999; 7:101.

De Smedt, T, de Jong, A, Van Leemput, W. Lateral epicondylitis in tennis: update on aetiology, biomechanics and treatment. Br J Sports Med 2007; 41:816.

Duffy, GP, Berry, DJ, Rowland, C, Cabanela, ME. Primary uncemented total hip arthroplasty in patients ≤40 years old: 10- to 14-year results using first-generation proximally porous-coated implants. J Arthroplasty 2001; 16:140.

Gordon, MD, Steiner, ME. Anterior Cruciate Ligament Injuries. In: Orthopaedic Knowledge Update Sports Medicine III, Garrick, JG, (Ed), American Academy of Orthopaedic Surgeons, Rosemont IL 2004; p.169.

Haahr, JP, Andersen, JH. Prognostic factors in lateral epicondylitis: a randomized trial with one-year follow-up in 266 new cases treated with minimal occupational intervention or the usual approach in general practice. Rheumatology (Oxford) 2003; 42:1216.

Jillapalli, D, Shefner, JM. Electrodiagnosis in common mononeuropathies and plexopathies. Semin Neurol 2005; 25:196.

Jones, IE, Williams, SM, Dow, N, Goulding, A. How many children remain fracture-free during growth? a longitudinal study of children and adolescents participating in the Dunedin Multidisciplinary Health and Development Study. Osteoporos Int 2002; 13:990.

Keir, PJ, Rempel, DM. Pathomechanics of peripheral nerve loading. Evidence in carpal tunnel syndrome. J Hand Ther 2005; 18:259.

Lavernia, CJ, Guzman, JF, Gachupin-Garcia, A. Cost effectiveness and quality of life in knee arthroplasty. Clin Orthop 1997 :134.

Linko, E, Harilainen, A, Malmivaara, A, Seitsalo, S. Surgical versus conservative interventions for anterior cruciate ligament ruptures in adults. Cochrane Database Syst Rev 2005 Apr 18;(2)

Khosla, S, Melton LJ, 3rd, Dekutoski, MB. Incidence of childhood distal forearm fractures over 30 years: a population-based study. JAMA 2003; 290:1479.

Kostogiannis, I, Ageberg, E, Neuman, P. Activity level and subjective knee function 15 years after anterior cruciate ligament injury: a prospective, longitudinal study of nonreconstructed patients. Am J Sports Med 2007; 35:1135.

Kujala, UM, Sarna, S, Kaprio, J. Cumulative incidence of achilles tendon rupture and tendinopathy in male former elite athletes. Clin J Sport Med 2005; 15:133.

Mayer, F, Hirschmuller, A, Muller, S. Effects of short-term treatment strategies over 4 weeks in Achilles tendinopathy. Br J Sports Med 2007; 41:e6.

Padua, L, Padua, R, Aprile, I. Multiperspective follow-up of untreated carpal tunnel syndrome: a multicenter study. Neurology 2001; 56:1459.

Perron, AD, Ingerski, MS, Brady, WJ. Acute complications associated with shoulder dislocation at an academic Emergency Department. J Emerg Med 2003; 24:141.

Peters-Veluthamaningal, C, van der, Windt DA, Winters, JC, Meyboom-de Jong, B. Corticosteroid injection for trigger finger in adults. Cochrane Database Syst Rev 2009; :CD005617.

Peters-Veluthamaningal, C, Winters, JC, Groenier, KH, Jong, BM. Corticosteroid injections effective for trigger finger in adults in general practice: a double-blinded randomised placebo controlled trial. Ann Rheum Dis 2008; 67:1262.

Priganc, VW, Henry, SM. The relationship among five common carpal tunnel syndrome tests and the severity of carpal tunnel syndrome. J Hand Ther 2003; 16:225.

Prodromos, CC, Han, Y, Rogowski, J. A meta-analysis of the incidence of anterior cruciate ligament tears as a function of gender, sport, and a knee injury-reduction regimen. Arthroscopy 2007; 23:1320.

Quam, JP, Michet, CJ Jr, Wilson, MG. Total knee arthroplasty: a population-based study. Mayo Clin Proc 1991; 66:589.

Saleh, KJ, Kassim, R, Yoon, P, Vorlicky, LN. Complications of total hip arthroplasty. Am J Orthop 2002; 31:485.

Schaider, J, Simon, RR. Shoulder Injuries. In: Clinical Practice of Emergency Medicine, Wolfson, AB, Hendey, GW, Hendry, PL, et al (Eds), Lippincott, Williams and Wilkins, Philadelphia 2005. p.1033.

Shiri, R, Viikari-Juntura, E, Varonen, H, Heliovaara, M. Prevalence and determinants of lateral and medial epicondylitis: a population study. Am J Epidemiol 2006; 164:1065.

Simon, RR, Sherman, SC, Koenigsknecht, SJ. Emergency Orthopedics: The Extremities, 5th ed, McGraw-Hill, New York 2006.

Sineff, SS, Reichman, EF. Shoulder Joint Dislocation Reduction. In: Emergency Medicine Procedures, Reichman, EF, Simon, RR, (Eds). McGraw-Hill, New York 2004. p.593.

Smidt, N, Lewis, M, VAN DER, Windt DA. Lateral epicondylitis in general practice: course and prognostic indicators of outcome. J Rheumatol 2006; 33:2053.

Struijs, PA, Kerkhoffs, GM, Assendelft, WJ, Van Dijk, CN. Conservative treatment of lateral epicondylitis: brace versus physical therapy or a combination of both-a randomized clinical trial. Am J Sports Med 2004; 32:462.

Suchak, AA, Bostick, G, Reid, D. The incidence of achilles tendon ruptures in Edmonton, Canada. Foot Ankle Int 2005; 26:932.

Wilson, MG, Kelley, K, Thornhill, TS. Infection as a complication of total knee-replacement arthroplasty. Risk factors and treatment in sixty-seven cases. J Bone Joint Surg Am 1990; 72:878.

Yang, K, Yeo, SJ, Lee, BP, Lo, NN. Total knee arthroplasty in diabetic patients: a study of 109 consecutive cases. J Arthroplasty 2001; 16:102.

Chapter 7: Neurosurgery

Adams HP Jr; del Zoppo G; Alberts MJ; Bhatt DL; Brass L., Guidelines for the early management of adults with ischemic stroke: a guideline from the American Heart Association/American Stroke Association Stroke Council, Clinical Cardiology Council, Cardiovascular Radiology and Intervention Council, and the Atherosclerotic Peripheral Vascular Disease and Quality of Care Outcomes in Research Interdisciplinary Working Groups: the American Academy of Neurology affirms the value of this guideline as an educational tool for neurologists. Stroke. 2007 May;38(5):1655-711. Epub 2007 Apr 12.

Armao D, Castillo M, Chen H,. "Colloid Cyst of the Third Ventricle: Imaging-pathologic Correlation. American Journal of NeuroRadiology 21:1470-1477, September 2000

Barker FG II, Jannetta PJ, Bissonette DJ. The long-term outcome of microvascular decompression for trigeminal neuralgia. New England Journal of Medicine 1996; 334: 1077-1083.

Benabid AL; Chabardes S; Mitrofanis J; Pollak P., Deep brain stimulation of the subthalamic nucleus for the treatment of Parkinson's disease. Department of Neurosurgery and Neurology, University of Grenoble, CHU Albert Michallon,

Grenoble,Lancet Neurol. 2009 Jan;8(1):67-81.

Chou R, Baisden J, Carragee EJ."Surgery for low back pain: a review of the evidence for an American Pain Society Clinical Practice Guideline". Spine (Phila Pa 1976) 2009 May 1;34(10):1094-109 Lippincott Williams & Wilkins

Chou R, Qaseem A. Diagnosis and treatment of low back pain: a joint clinical practice guideline from the American College of Physicians and the American Pain Society. Ann Intern Med. 2007;147(7):478-491.

Dennis MS; Bamford JM; Sandercock PA; Warlow CP., A comparison of risk factors and prognosis for transient ischemic attacks and minor ischemic strokes. The Oxfordshire Community Stroke Project. Stroke 1989 Nov;20(11):1494-9.

Duane E Haines. Neuroanatomy: An Atlas of Structures, Sections and Systems, 7th Ed.

Eskandar EN, Cosgrove GR, Shinobu L. Surgery for Parkinson's Disease. http://neurosurgery.mgh.harvard.edu/functional/PDsurgery.htm. Accessed June 28, 2010.

Fauci, Braunwald, Kasper Harrison's: Principal of Internal Medicine, 17th Ed Chapter 336 pp2583-2587, pp2605-7, pp2549-2559

Lawrence M. Brass, M.D. Yale University School of medicine heart book. Chapter 18 Stroke.

Marosi C; Hassler M; Roessler K; Reni M; Sant M; Mazza E; Vecht C., Meningioma. Crit Rev Oncol Hematol. 2008 Aug;67(2):153-71. Epub 2008 Mar 14.

Mathews MS, Sharma J, Snyder KV, Natarajan SK, Siddiqui AH, Hopkins LN, Levy EI. Safety, effectiveness, and practicality of endovascular therapy within the first 3 hours of acute ischemic stroke onset. Neurosurgery. 2009 Nov;65(5):860-5.

NASCET Investigators. North American Symptomatic Carotid Endarterectomy Trial: methods, patient characteristics, and progress. Stroke 1991;22:711-20.Neurology 2003; 60: E3-E5; American Academy of Neurology

Neurological Sciences, London Health Sciences Centre, London, Ontario, Canada. Brain 2005 May;128(Pt 5):1188-98. Epub 2005 Mar 9.Schiff, D, Hsu, L, Wen, PY. Uncommon brain tumors, skull base tumors, and intracranial cysts. In: Office Practice of Neurology, Samuels, MA, Feske, S. (Eds)., 2nd edition. Churchill Livingstone, New York, 2003. p.1092.

OHSU Brain Institute - Disease Statistics. http://www.ohsu.edu/xd/education/schools/
research-institutes/brain-institute/about/disease-statistics.cfm. Accessed June 28,
2010.

Osterman H; Seitsalo S; Karppinen J; Malmivaara A., Effectiveness of microdiscectomy
for lumbar disc herniation: a randomized controlled trial with 2 years of follow-up.
Spine. 2006 Oct 1;31(21):2409-14.

Schankin CJ; Gall C; Straube A., Headache syndromes after acoustic neuroma surgery
and their implications for quality of life. Cephalalgia. 2009 Jul;29(7):760-71. Epub
2009 Feb 23.

Schroder HW, Gaab MR,. "Endoscopic resection of colloid cysts" Department of
Neurosurgery, Ernst Mortiz Arndt Univ, Germany. 2002 Dec;51(6):1441-4

Spencer SS; Berg AT; Vickrey BG; Sperling MR; Bazil CW; Shinnar S; Langfitt JT; Walczak
TS; Pacia., Predicting long-term seizure outcome after resective epilepsy surgery:
the multicenter study. Department of Neurology, Yale University School of Medicine.
Neurology 2005 Sep 27;65(6):912-8.

Tellez-Zenteno JF; Dhar R; Wiebe S., Long-term seizure outcomes following epilepsy
surgery: a systematic review and meta-analysis. Department of Clinical

Weaver F; Follett K; Hur K; Ippolito D; Stern M., Deep brain stimulation in Parkinson
disease: a metaanalysis of patient outcomes. Midwest Center for Health Services. J
Neurosurg. 2005 Dec;103(6):956-67.

Weinstein JN; Tosteson TD; Lurie JD; Tosteson AN., Surgical versus nonsurgical therapy
for lumbar spinal stenosis. Dartmouth Institute for Health Policy and Clinical Practice,
Department of Orthopedics, Dartmouth Medical School.

Xu WX, Lu D, Wang J,. "Surgical treatment of the old with degenerative lumbar spinal
stenosis". Zhongguo Gu Shang. 2010 Apr;23(4):261-3

Yano S; Kuratsu J., Indications for surgery in patients with asymptomatic meningiomas
based on an extensive experience. Department of Neurosurgery, Faculty of Medical
and Pharmaceutical Sciences, Kumamoto University Graduate School, Kumamoto,
Japan. J Neurosurg. 2006 Oct;105(4):538-43.

Chapter 8: Plastic Surgery

American Society of Aesthetic Plastic Surgeons. (n.d.). American Society of Aesthetic Plastic Surgeons. Retrieved June 15, 2010, from American Society of Aesthetic Plastic Surgeons: www.surgery.org

American Society of Plastic Surgeons and American Society for Aesthetic Plastic Surgeons. (2000, February 12). Policy statement on accreditation of office facilities. Retrieved June 15, 2010, from American Society of Plastic Surgeons: www.plasticsurgery.org

Atiyeh, B. R. (2008). Aesthetic/cosmetic surgery and ethical challenges. Aesthetic Plastic Surgery , 32, 829-839.

Botney, R. (2008). Improving patient safety in anesthesia: A success story? Int. J Radiat Oncol Biol Phys , 71, S182.

Camp, M. W. (2010). Who is providing aesthetic surgery? A detailed examination of the geographic distribution and training backgrounds of cosmetic practitioners in southern California. Plastic and Reconstructive Surgery , 125, 1257-1262.

Cinella, G. M. (2007). Sedation analgesia during office-based plastic surgery procedures: Comparison of two opiod regimines. Plastic and Reconstructive Surgery , 2263-2270.

D'Amico, R. S. (2008, May). Risks and opportunities for plastic surgeons in a widening cosmetic medicine market: Future demand, consumer preferences, and trends in practitioners' services. Plastic and Reconstructive Surgery , 1787-1792.

Habbema, L. (2009). Safety of liposuction using exclusively tumescent local anesthesia in 3,240 consecutive cases. Dermatol. Surg. , 35, 1728-1735.

Hasen, K. S. (2003). An outcome study comparing intravenous sedation with midazolam/fentanyl (conscious sedation) versus propofol infusion (deep sedation) for aesthetic surgery. Plastic and Reconstructive Surgery , 1683-1689.

Hughes C.E. III. (2001). Reduction of lipoplasty risks and mortality: An ASAPS survey. Aesthetic Surgery Journal , 21, 120-127.

Iverson, R. L. (2004). American Society of Plastic Surgeons Committee on Patient Safety. Practice advisory on liposuction. Plastic and Reconstructive Surgery , 1478-1490.

Lanier, W. (2006). A three-decade perspective on anesthesia safety. Am Surg , 72, 985.

Morello, D. C. (1997). Patient safety in accredited office surgical facilities. Plastic and Reconstructive Surgery , 1496.

Plastic Surgery Information Service. (2000, June 24). What you should know about the safety of outpatient plastic surgery. Retrieved June 15, 2010, from American Society of Plastic Surgeons: www.plasticsurgery.org

Rao, R. E. (1999). Deaths related to liposuction. New England Journal of Medicine , 340, 1471-1475.

Rohrich, R. B. (1999). Is liposuction safe? Plastic and Reconstructive Surgery , 104, 819.

Rohrich, R. W. (2001). Safety of Outpatient Surgery: Is Mandatory Accreditation of Outpatient Surgery Centers Enough? Plastic and Reconstructive Surgery , 107 (1), 189-192.

TA, N. (1993). Ambulatory office general anesthesia. In Anesthesia for Facial Plastic Surgery. New York: Thieme Medicall Publishers.

Task Force on Sedation and Analgesia by Non-Anesthesiologists. (2002). Practice guidelines for sedation and analgesia by non-anesthesiologists: an updated report by the American Society of Anesthesiologists Task Force on Sedation and Analgesia by Non-Anesthesiologists. Anesthesiology , 1004.

Taub, P. B. (2010). Anesthesia for cosmetic surgery. Plastic and Reconstructive Surgery , 125 (1), 1e-7e.

The American Society of Plastic Surgeons. (2009). Find a Surgeon. Retrieved June 15, 2010, from The American Society of Plastic Surgeons: www.plasticsurgery.org/ebusiness4/PatientConsumers/findasurgeon.aspx

USA Today. (2000, August 23). Slow down office surgeries. USA Today .

Whitaker, I. K. (2007). The birth of plastic surgery: The story of nasal reconstruction from the Edwin Smith Papyrus to the twenty-first century. Plastic and Reconstructive Surgery , 120, 327-336.

White PF, F. A. (2005). Ambulatory (outpatient) anesthesia. In M. RD, Miller's Anesthesia, 6th ed. (pp. 2589-2635). Philadelphia, PA: Elsevier Churchill Livingstone.

Wolters, U. W. (1996). ASA classification and perioperative variables as predictors of postoperative outcome. Br J Anaesth , 77, 217.

Yoon, H. Y. (2002). Low-dose propofol infusion for sedation during local anesthesia. Plastic and Reconstructive Surgery , 956.

Youn, A. (2005). The Yellow Pages plastic surgeon. Plastic and Reconstructive Surgery , 115, 317-319.

Chapter 9: Urology

Addanki K., Pace D., Bagasra O., "A practice for all seasons: male circumcision and the prevention of HIV transmission" Journal of Infectious Developing Countries 2008; 2(5): 328-334

American Cancer Society. Cancer Facts and Figures 2008. Atlanta, Ga, USA: American Cancer Society; 2008.

Chang HC, Chen SC, Chen J, Hsieh JT. "Initial 10-year experience of sperm cryopreservation services for cancer patients." J Formos Med Assoc. 2006 Dec;105(12):1022-6.

Donoval B., Landay A., Moses A., "HIV-1 target cells in foreskins of African men with varying histories of sexually transmitted infections". American Journal of Clinical Pathology 2006 Mar;125(3):386-91.

Dhar N., Jones J., "Vasectomy: A simple snip?" Indian Journal of Urology. 2007. Vol.23 (1) 6-8

Eberhard J., Stahl O., Cwikiel M., "Risk factors for post-treatment hypogonadism in testicular cancer patients" Department of Oncology, Lund Hospital, Sweden. European Journal of Endocrinology 2008 April;158(4):561-70.

Enciso M., Muriel L., Fernandez J.,"Infertile Men with Varicocele show a High Relative Proportion of Sperm cells with Intense Nuclear Damage Level, Evidenced by the Sperm Chromatin Dispersion Test. "Journal of Andrology, Vol. 27, No.1 Jan/Feb 2006

Esteves S., Glina S., "Recovery of Spermatogenesis after microsurgical subinguinal varicocele in azoospermic men based on testicular histology". International Brazilian Journal of Urology. 2005;31:541-8

Fauci, Braunwald, Kasper. "Harrison's Principles of Internal Medicine 17th Ed."Chapter

340 pp.2310-2324

Gingell C., Carroll R., "Review of the complications and medico legal implications of vasectomy". Postgraduate medical Journal 2001; 77 656-659.

Gupta NP., Kolla SB., Seth A., "Radical cystectomy for bladder cancer: A single center experience". Indian Journal of Urology. 2008 Jan;24(1):54-9

Hall P., "Nephrolithiasis: Treatment, causes and prevention" Cleveland Clinic Journal of Medicine October 2009 vol.76 sup.10 p583-591

Heilberg I., Schor N., "Renal stone disease: causes, evaluation and medical treatment" Division of Nephrology, University of San Paulo, San Paulo Brazil. 2006

Hellstrom W., Bivalacqua T., "Peyronie's Disease: Etiology, medical, and surgical therapy". Journal of Andrology, Vol.21, No.3 May/June 2000.

Hsueh Po-Ren, "Human papillomavirus, genital warts and vaccines" Journal of Microbiology and Immunology and Infections. 2009;42:101-106.

Huang CM., "Human papillomavirus and vaccination". Mayo Clinic Proceedings". June 2008 Vol.83 No.6 701-707.

Jalkut M., Cadavid N., Rajfer J., "Peyronie's Disease: A review". Dept. of Urology, UCLA. Reviews in Urology. 2003 Summer; 5(3):142-148.

Jemal A, Siegel R, Ward E, Hao Y, Xu J, Thun MJ. Cancer statistics. CA Cancer J Clin ; 2009;59:225–49.

Jiang X., Yaun J., Skipper P., "Environmental Tobacco Smoke and Bladder Cancer risk in never smokers of Los Angeles County" Cancer Research. Aug. 1, 2007 67;7540

Kamischke A, Jürgens H, Hertle L, Berdel WE, Nieschlag E. "Cryopreservation of sperm from adolescents and adults with malignancies." J Androl. 2004 Jul-Aug;25(4):586-92.

Leman E., Gonzalgo M., "Prognostic features and markers for testicular cancer management". Indian Journal of Urology 2010 Jan-Mar; 26(1):76-81

Levy A., Smaraj G., "Benign prostatic hyperplasia: When to 'watch and wait', when and how to treat. Cleveland Clinic Journal of Medicine Vol.74-Sup.3 May 2007.

Maddineni S., Lau M., Sangar V., " Identifying the needs of penile cancer suffers: A systematic review of the quality of life, psychosexual and psychosocial literature in penile cancer". BMC Urology. 2009; 9:8.

Miller N., Lingeman E., "Management of kidney stones" Methodist Hosp Institute for Kidney Disease, Indiana University. BMJ 2007; 334:468-472

Mohseni MG., Zand S., Aghamir SMK., "Effect of smoking on prognosistic factors of Transitional Cell Carcinoma of the Bladder". Urology Journal. Autumn 2004 Vol. 1 No.4 pp250-252

Moses S.,"Male circumcision: a new approach to reducing HIV transmission". CMAJ. 2009 October 13; 181(8): E134-E135

Romero FR, Romero KR, Mattos MA, Garcia CR, Fernandes RC, Perez MD. Sexual function after partial penectomy for penile cancer. Urology. 2005; 66:1292–5.

Sandhu J., "Therapeutic options in the treatment of benign prostatic hyperplasia" Patient Prefer Adherence. 2009; 3: 213-223.

Silber S., Grotjan E., "Microscopic Vasectomy Reversal 30 years later: A summary of 4010 cases by the same surgeon". Journal of Andrology, Vol.25, No.6, Nov./Dec. 2004.

Tobian AA, Serwadda D, Quinn TC, Kigozi G, Gravitt PE, Laeyendecker O, Charvat B, Ssempijja V, Riedesel M, Oliver AE, Nowak RG, Moulton LH, Chen MZ, Reynolds SJ, Wawer MJ, Gray RH. Male circumcision for the prevention of HSV-2 and HPV infections and syphilis. N Engl J Med. 2009 Mar 26;360(13):1298-309.

Windahl T, Skeppner E, Andersson SO, Fugl-Meyer KS. Sexual function and satisfaction in men aftor laser treatment for penile carcinoma. J Urol. 2004; 172:648–51.

Zini A., Blumenfeld A., Libman J., Willis J., "Beneficial effect of microsurgical varicocelectomy on human sperm DNA integrity". Division of Urology, St. Mary's Hosp. McGill University., Oxford Journals-Human Reproduction. 2005 Apr;20(4):1018-21

Chapter 10: Ophthalmology: Eye Surgery

Agency for Healthcare Research and Quality. Evidence Report/Technology Assessment: Number 16. Anesthesia management during cataract surgery. Washington, DC: AHRQ Publication No. 00-E015; 2000. Available at: http://www.ahrq.gov/clinic/epcsums/

anestsum.htm. Accessed July 6, 2010.

American Academy of Ophthalmology and American Society of Cataract and Refractive Surgery Joint Position Statement. Ophthalmic Postoperative Care. San Francisco: American Academy of Ophthalmology, 2000. Available at: http://www.aao.org/education/statements. Accessed July 6, 2010.

AmericanAcademy of Ophthalmology Refractive Management/Intervention Panel. Preferred Practice Pattern®Guidelines. Refractive Errors & Refractive Surgery. San Francisco, CA: AmericanAcademy of Ophthalmology; 2007. Available at: http://www. aao.org/ppp. Accessed July 7, 2010.

Argento C, Fernandez Mendy J, Cosentino MJ. Laser in situ keratomileusis versus arcuate keratotomy to treat astigmatism. J Cataract Refract Surg 1999;25:374-82.

Baikoff G, Matach G, Fontaine A. Correction of presbyopia with refractive multifocal phakic intraocular lenses. J Cataract Refract Surg 2004;30:1454-60.

Boezaart A, Berry R, Nell M. "Topical Anesthesia Verses Retrobulbar Block for Cataract Surgery: The Patient's Perspective." J Clin Anesth. 2000; 12:58-6.

Bosniak S. Reconstructive upper lid blepharoplasty. Ophthalmol Clin North Am. Jun 2005; 18(2): 279-89, vi.

Burr JM, Mowatt G, Hernández R, Siddiqui MA, Cook J, Lourenco T. The clinical effectiveness and cost-effectiveness of screening for open angle glaucoma: a systematic review and economic evaluation. Health Technol Assess. 2007 Oct;11(41):iii-iv, ix-x, 1-190.

Cobp-Soriano R, Calvo MA, Beltran J, Llovet FL, Baviera J. J Cataract Refract Surg. 2005 Jul;31(7):1357-65.IG.Thin flap laser in situ keratomileusis: analysis of contrast sensitivity, visual, and refractive outcomes.

Duffey RJ, Leaming D. US trends in refractive surgery: 2003 ISRS/AAO survey. J Refract Surg. 2005 Jan-Feb;21(1):87-91.

Feinberg, Edward B. "Cataract: MedlinePlus Medical Encyclopedia." National Library of Medicine - National Institutes of Health. http://www.nlm.nih.gov/medlineplus/ency/article/001001.htm. Accessed July 8, 2010.

Griggs, Paul B. "LASIK Eye Surgery: MedlinePlus Medical Encyclopedia." National Library of Medicine - National Institutes of Health. http://www.nlm.nih.gov/medlineplus/ency/

article/007018.htm. Accessed July 6, 2010.

Griggs, Paul B. "Refractive Corneal Surgery - Discharge: MedlinePlus Medical Encyclopedia." National Library of Medicine - National Institutes of Health. http://www.nlm.nih.gov/medlineplus/ency/patientinstructions/000245.htm. Accessed July 6, 2010.

Hersh PS, Steinert RF, Brint SF. Photorefractive keratectomy versus laser in situ keratomileusis: comparison of optical side effects. Summit PRK-LASIK Study Group. Ophthalmology. May 2000;107(5):925-33.

Hoenig JA. Comprehensive management of eyebrow and forehead ptosis. Otolaryngol Clin North Am. Oct 2005; 38(5): 947-84.

Kwon YH, Figert JH, Kuehn MH, Alward WL. Primary open-angle glaucoma. N Engl J Med. 2009 Mar 12;360(11):1113-24.

McGhee CN, Craig JP, Sachdev N, Weed KH, Brown AD. Functional, psychological and satisfaction outcomes of laser in situ keratomileusis for high myopia. J Cataract Refract Surg 2000 Apr;26(4):497-509.

Migdal C. Glaucoma medical treatment: philosophy, principles and practice. Eye. Jun 2000;14 (Pt 3B):515-8.

Nettina, Sandra. Lippincott Manual of Nursing Practicing, 7th edition. Philadelphia: Lippincot, 2001, pp. 115-117.

Piltz-Seymour JR. Does Your Patient Have Glaucoma?. Review of Ophthalmol. 1999;VI(6):86-99.

Roque, Manolette R., Barbara L. Roque, Ruben Limbonsiong, and Roberto II Pineda. "Hyperopia and Presbyopia, Conductive Keratoplasty: EMedicine Ophthalmology." EMedicine - Medical Reference. 24 Oct. 2008. http://emedicine.medscape.com/article/1222433-overview. Accessed July 6, 2010.

Rowsey J. Review: Current concepts in astigmatism surgery. J Refract Surg 1986;2:85-94.

Schallhorn SC. Avoidance, recognition, and management of LASIK complications. Am J Ophthalmol. Apr 2006; 141(4): 733-9.

Shortt AJ, Allan BD. Photorefractive keratectomy (PRK) versus laser-assisted in-situ keratomileusis (LASIK) for myopia. Cochrane Database Syst Rev 2006:CD005135.

US Food and Drug Administration: Center for Devices and Radiological Health. Lasik eye surgery. Updated September 22, 2009.

Vass C, Hirn C, Sycha T, Findl O, Bauer P, Schmetterer L. Medical interventions for primary open angle glaucoma and ocular hypertension. Cochrane Database Syst Rev. 2007 Oct 17;(4)

"What Should I Expect Before, During, and after Surgery?" U S Food and Drug Administration Home Page. Web. June 2010. http://www.fda.gov/MedicalDevices/ ProductsandMedicalProcedures/SurgeryandLifeSupport/LASIK/ucm061270.htm. Accessed July 10, 2010.

Chapter 11: Interventional Radiology

Abrams, Herbert L. "Abrams' angiography: interventional radiology" 2nd ed. Philadelphia: Lippincott Williams & Wilkins, 2006.

American College of Radiology www.acr.org Accessed July 2010

Baylor College of Medicine "Uterine Fibroid Embolization" http://www. debakeydepartmentofsurgery.org/home/content.cfm?proc_name=Uterine+Fibroid+E mbolization&content_id=272 2008 Accessed July 2010

BlueCross BlueShield of Alabama "Get Wise About Radiation Exposure from CT Scans" https://www.bcbsal.org/health/important/CTScans.pdf. Accessed July 18, 2010

Ferrucci, Joseph T "Interventional radiology of the abdomen" Baltimore: Williams & Wilkins, 1985.

Health Physics Society "Radiation Exposure from Medical Diagnostic Imaging Procedures" http://www.hps.org/documents/meddiagimaging.pdf. Accessed July 18, 2010

Kaufman, John A. "Vascular and interventional radiology" 1st ed. St. Louis: Mosby, 2004.

McGraw, J. Kevin "Interventional radiology of the spine" Totowa, N.J.: Humana Press, 2004.

Radiology Info.org "Safety: Radiation Exposure in X-ray Examinations" http://www. radiologyinfo.org/en/pdf/sfty_xray.pdf. Accessed July 21, 2010

Radiology Info.org "Uterine Fibroid Embolization" http://www.radiologyinfo.org/en/info.
cfm?pg=ufe. Accessed July 16, 2010.

Siddiqi, Nasir H. "Contrast Medium Reactions, Recognition and Treatment" http://
emedicine.medscape.com/article/422855-overview 2009

Siskin, Gary P. "Interventional radiology in women's health" New York: Thieme, 2009.

Siskin, Gary P. "Uterine Fibroid Embolization" http://emedicine.medscape.com/
article/421734-overview. Accessed July 16, 2010.

Thomsen, H.S., Morcos, S.K. "Contrast media and the kidney: European Society of
Urogenital Radiology (ESUR) Guidelines" British Journal of Radiology (2003) 76,
513-518

Topol, Eric J. Textbook of interventional cardiology" Philadelphia: Saunders/Elsevier, 2008.

Valji, Karim. "Vascular and Interventional Radiology" Philadelphia: Saunders, 1999.

Wolanske, Kirsten. Gordon, Sze. "Uterine Artery Embolization" Applied Radiology.
2004;33(10) © 2004

World Health Organization. "Efficacy and radiation safety in interventional radiology" 2000.

www.ingramcontent.com/pod-product-compliance
Lightning Source LLC
Chambersburg PA
CBHW051518170526
45165CB00002B/517

* 9 7 8 1 4 5 3 6 9 1 3 7 3 *